August 25 Four weeks

The plastic test stick has two lines.

I should be thrilled. I wanted this. I try to imagine holding a tiny baby in my arms. Awestruck. But my thoughts quickly turn to all those other sticks with two lines, all the thwarted promise. My stomach churns, and it's hard to breathe.

I stare at myself in the mirror above the sink, blond hair starting to gray, blue eyes tired, fair skin pasty. Am I ready for this? What if I lose another baby? I open the bathroom door. Jon waits, hazel eyes wide, lips parted. His breath sputters, still labored from a ten-mile run. "Okay." I nod. "Here we go."

—from *To Full Term*

Gabra—
Good luck
with your writing!
Darci Kl—

TO FULL TERM

A Mother's Triumph Over Miscarriage

DARCI KLEIN

Foreword by
MARY STEPHENSON, M.D., M.Sc.

BERKLEY BOOKS, NEW YORK

THE BERKLEY PUBLISHING GROUP
Published by the Penguin Group
Penguin Group (USA) Inc.
375 Hudson Street, New York, New York 10014, USA
Penguin Group (Canada), 90 Eglinton Avenue East, Suite 700, Toronto, Ontario M4P 2Y3, Canada
(a division of Pearson Penguin Canada Inc.)
Penguin Books Ltd., 80 Strand, London WC2R 0RL, England
Penguin Group Ireland, 25 St. Stephen's Green, Dublin 2, Ireland (a division of Penguin Books Ltd.)
Penguin Group (Australia), 250 Camberwell Road, Camberwell, Victoria 3124, Australia
(a division of Pearson Australia Group Pty. Ltd.)
Penguin Books India Pvt. Ltd., 11 Community Centre, Panchsheel Park, New Delhi—110 017, India
Penguin Group (NZ), 67 Apollo Drive, Rosedale, North Shore 0745, Auckland, New Zealand
(a division of Pearson New Zealand Ltd.)
Penguin Books (South Africa) (Pty.) Ltd., 24 Sturdee Avenue, Rosebank, Johannesburg 2196,
South Africa

Penguin Books Ltd., Registered Offices: 80 Strand, London WC2R 0RL, England

This book is an original publication of The Berkley Publishing Group.

PRINTING HISTORY
Berkley trade paperback edition / June 2007

Library of Congress Cataloging-in-Publication Data

Klein, Darci.
    To full term : a mother's triumph over miscarriage / Darci Klein ; foreword by Mary Stephenson.
    p. cm.
    Includes bibliographical references.
    ISBN 978-0-425-21587-6
    1. Klein, Darci—Health. 2. Miscarriage—Patients—United States—Biography. 3. Pregnant women—
United States—Biography. I. Title.

    RG648.K53   2007
    618.3'920092—dc22
    [B]   2007006427

PRINTED IN THE UNITED STATES OF AMERICA

10 9 8 7 6 5 4 3 2 1

PUBLISHER'S NOTE:
All events depicted in this book are real, although some of the names and details have been changed to
protect privacy. All of the doctors' names have been changed.

Every effort has been made to ensure that the information contained in this book is complete and accurate. However, neither the publisher nor the author is engaged in rendering professional advice or ser-
vices to the individual reader. The ideas, procedures, and suggestions contained in this book are not
intended as a substitute for consulting with your physician. All matters regarding your health require
medical supervision. Neither the author nor the publisher shall be liable or responsible for any loss or
damage allegedly arising from any information or suggestion in this book.

While the author has made every effort to provide accurate telephone numbers and Internet addresses at
the time of publication, neither the publisher nor the author assumes any responsibility for errors, or for
changes that occur after publication. Further, the publisher does not have any control over and does not
assume any responsibility for author or third-party websites or their content.

For M and E

ACKNOWLEDGMENTS

I'd like to thank the people who shared their love, wisdom, and support while I wrote this book, and during my pregnancy with Sam.

First, my husband, Jon, for his authentic love, generous encouragement, and unshakable belief in my ability to write this book. Thank you, sweetheart. I am immensely grateful for my wondrous children, Maddie and Sam, for their love and inspiration, and for making me appreciate the privilege of motherhood. I also send love and gratitude to Steve and Evelyn Klein for their unmatched enthusiasm, always available ears, and endless devotion. I simply adore you both. And I'm filled with the deepest appreciation for Deborah Paver, Stacy Tarbis, and Kelly Masjoan, women who lift me with the mere sound of their voices. I love you all. Completely.

I would also like to thank Lisa Gal, Kelly Masjoan, Rob Erlichman, and Alice Wang for their thoughtful review of my manuscript. Your feedback made this a better book. And I am enormously appreciative of Dr. Mary Stephenson for all her time spent writing the foreword, and along with Dr. Jonathan Scher, providing rich insights into the mysteries of obstetrics and delivering essential feedback about my manuscript. I also owe thanks to Dr. Alan Beer, a dedicated physician who shaped the way I think about the problem of pregnancy loss.

I am deeply grateful to my agent, Sorche Fairbank, and my editor, Samantha Mandor. Both women have been true partners in this endeavor, providing insightful input and unwavering belief in the need for this book. My sincere thanks to the rest of my supporters at Penguin: Leslie Schwartz, Susan Allison, Denise Silvestro, and Leslie Gelbman, for their commitment to get this book into the hands of families who have suffered loss. And reverent thanks to Margo Perin and Lara JK Wilson, wise and inspirational women who helped develop my writing, and to Grub Street for building a real community for Boston writers.

And finally, I feel infinite gratitude toward those who cared for me during my pregnancy with Sam: my Boston obstetricians whose diligent care kept us both safe, my beloved friend Mary Fuller for her sincere friendship, and our many neighbors whose gourmet meals sustained our family both physically and spiritually.

FOREWORD

No pregnancy loss should go unnoticed. Whether it occurs a few days before or after a missed period, at eight weeks or at eight months, each pregnancy loss is devastating in its own way, with the dreams of the future disappearing in a moment. Unfortunately, as a woman experiences more and more pregnancy losses, instead of being supported, she often becomes isolated; first from friends, then family, and sometimes from her partner. I often hear a patient say, "I didn't tell my partner because I didn't want to hurt him." Such isolation can lead to unresolved grief, anxiety, depression, and worse. Conversely, with an ongoing pregnancy, such patients may have developed defense mechanisms to ease their pain that can impede bonding during the antenatal course and following delivery. Although it is difficult, breaking down the barriers and thinking about "having a baby" is necessary after experiencing a devastating pregnancy loss or losses. And even after a successful pregnancy outcome, some patients return to ask, "What if?" and "Why didn't I have this treatment last time?"—questions that usually remain un-answered.

Not all women overcome their history of recurrent preg-nancy loss. *To Full Term* illustrates how one person, Darci Klein, took control of what she could in order to optimize her likeli-hood of having another child. Her sadness, frustration, and over-whelming desire to try again led her to review the literature and try to figure out why her pregnancy losses occurred. She focused on the published research, asked questions, and sought out physicians who were receptive to her approach. She tells an amazing story of her drive to make sure she did everything she could to prevent another pregnancy loss, while balancing her role as a mother, wife, and working woman.

As director of a recurrent pregnancy loss program since 1992, first in Vancouver, Canada, and now at the University of Chicago, I have evaluated thousands of women and their partners who have experienced pregnancy loss. Each patient and her history of recurrent pregnancy loss is unique, influenced by her social and personal situation. Concomitant difficulties of conceiving and the impact of advancing maternal age complicate the evaluation and management. Cultural pressures can greatly influence how the patient and her partner discuss their history of recurrent pregnancy loss and how they will proceed with another preg-nancy attempt. It is not a matter of completing an evaluation for recurrent pregnancy loss; the societal, cultural, and personal pres-sures must be addressed to optimize management of a subse-quent pregnancy. Even with all of these issues addressed, some women will lose another pregnancy, but hopefully the sadness will be manageable with the assistance of family and friends.

Statistics show that more than two million women in the United States will have a pregnancy loss each year, a conservative estimate because pregnancies are not reported and many are passed at home without intervention. Ninety-five percent of pregnancy losses occur before ten weeks of gestation, most commonly due to a random error of early cell division in the oocyte or sperm, resulting in an extra chromosome, an absent chromosome, or an extra set of chromosomes. Research shows that an abnormality in the number of chromosomes accounts for about 50 percent of miscarriages prior to ten weeks of gestation. But the critical question is: Which miscarriages are random and which are not? Only by sending the miscarriage for chromosome testing can this be determined, a practice that is not universally embraced in this country. Women and their partners need answers to deal with their grief and to make an informed decision about whether to try again. Physicians need answers as well, to guide us in the evaluation and management of subsequent pregnancies. Chromosome testing of miscarriages is a pivotal part of evaluating recurrent pregnancy loss. Hopefully, with this book and others, such testing will increase in this country and abroad.

I have spent much of my career lecturing about recurrent pregnancy loss, building awareness of this common reproductive problem, teaching physicians how to identify which patients require evaluation beyond chromosome testing of the miscarriage and which do not. Unfortunately, our society minimizes the significance of miscarriage. This needs to change so that women and their partners will be evaluated sooner, scientifically proven treatments will be offered, and supportive, close monitoring will be the norm. All of these measures will result in improved live birthrates of couples with a history of fetal demise or recurrent pregnancy loss. The emotional toll associated with pregnancy loss is huge; patients need time, evidence-based medical care, and support to break away from its spiraling downward impact. Even after a successful pregnancy, the shadow of what was lost can linger for years to come.

I remember Darci walking into my office in 2005, telling me her story of a premature birth, early miscarriages, and the late loss of twins. This was followed by a list of questions reflecting her depth of investigation into why three of her pregnancies were not successful. Darci's story is not unique; it happens to many women in our country, but unfortunately it often is not talked about. A commitment to make change, as Darci has illustrated, will increase awareness of the issues and the impact of pregnancy loss in our society. Heightened awareness and lobbying for increased research funding will improve our knowledge and management for women and their partners who suffer from this frequent reproductive problem. Presently, our medical management is often "hypotheses driven," unsupported by properly designed trials to determine whether treatment is effective. This needs to change, so that women are offered effective and safe treatment to prevent pregnancy loss.

Darci concluded in her book that medical care after pregnancy loss is often inadequate, leaving many women to lose subsequent pregnancies that could have been saved with appropriate testing of the miscarriage. She wanted to know if I agreed with her conclusion. I do.

Mary D. Stephenson, M.D., M.Sc.,
professor and director of the Recurrent Pregnancy Loss Program
University of Chicago, Department of Obstetrics and Gynecology
Chicago, Illinois

INTRODUCTION

I did not want to write this book.

After the torture of watching my premature daughter struggle for seven weeks in a neonatal intensive care unit (NICU), the anguish of two miscarriages, and then the devastation of giving birth to twins at twenty weeks gestation, I wanted to believe that my crushing experience was rare, that losses like mine were an anomaly in a country with such advanced medical care.

But I am not an anomaly. Countless women have histories just as tragic as mine. And the medical community could have prevented many of our losses—but they didn't. Women need to know this. I need to tell them.

Pregnancy loss is a pervasive problem that leaves women feeling crushed and desolate. More than two million women lose pregnancies in this country every year. These women grieve, longing for the child that almost was, battling the depression and anxiety that often follows miscarriage. Their anguish can be intensified if partners cannot understand their grief, making women feel alone at a time when support is essential. And whether this is a first loss or a fifth, many families are at risk for future miscarriages, further tragedies that could be prevented with basic diagnostic tests after pregnancy loss.

Mainstream obstetricians do not treat pregnancy loss as a medical disorder that warrants diagnosis and preventive treatment. According to standard medical guidelines, obstetricians should withhold tests to investigate causes of loss until *two or more* consecutive miscarriages, giving doctors complete discretion on whether women get testing. The result? Some doctors test patients after two losses; others don't test patients until four or five losses. And because patients don't know about these guidelines, they do not realize that tests have been forgone—evaluations that could have detected treatable disorders before more pregnancies were lost, saving babies that will instead succumb to the systematic deficiencies in obstetric care.

At least seven hundred thousand pregnancies are lost to treatable disorders every year. This is the unspoken secret within a medical community that rarely offers even basic diagnostic testing after pregnancy loss. The accepted guideline that tells doctors to withhold testing until *multiple consecutive miscarriages* relies on the established finding that half of all losses are caused by chromosome abnormalities, and are thus unavoidable and untreatable. This guideline ignores the inalienable logic within this conventional wisdom: *The other half are not caused by chromosome abnormalities.*

When women lose chromosomally normal babies and are thoroughly tested for causes of loss, at least 60 percent have a treatable disorder. Recent advances likely push this number even higher. With treatment, most of these women can have a successful pregnancy. Without treatment, many will relive the tragedy of miscarriage.

I wrote this book because of the lesson I learned after my own losses: Most women will not get adequate diagnostic care after pregnancy loss unless they demand thorough testing. But because we have been conditioned to defer to physicians, many women are reluctant to make demands of their doctors. When speaking with an obstetrician after pregnancy loss, women must overcome this cultural norm and ask for a comprehensive evaluation.

After my last loss, twins at twenty weeks, I had little faith in the doctors who had previously done a few tests and erroneously said nothing was awry. I got more involved in my own care, leveraging my background as a career market researcher with an education in statistics, to investigate causes of loss. I insisted on a wider range of tests than doctors had offered, and soon had a longer list of test results to share with specialists.

I saw four physicians, asking each only one question: Why did I lose my babies? Even with all the diagnostics, none could answer with certainty; they offered theories, mere opinion on a literal matter of life and death. Obstetricians are often reduced to speculation when diagnosing causes of pregnancy loss, a reality fueled by the dearth of dollars spent toward researching causes of miscarriage. The National Institutes of Health, the largest provider of research funding, spends so little investigating miscarriage that it doesn't even publicly report the number.[1]

I was eventually diagnosed with cervical incompetence, the leading cause of late loss, and Factor V Leiden, a recently uncovered clotting disorder that affects more than ten million women in the United States alone, or roughly 6 percent of the female population. Both of these conditions are fairly common, but rarely diagnosed.

Physicians seldom diagnose cervical incompetence before women have endured the horror of multiple late losses. And few mainstream doctors diagnose Factor V Leiden—despite its prevalence—because sluggish obstetric guidelines that have not been revised since 2001 do not yet recognize this treatable disorder as a cause of pregnancy loss. Despite fourteen credible studies that say Factor V Leiden can cause pregnancy loss, obstetric guidelines tell doctors not to perform this test when seeking the cause of early recurrent miscarriage.

I was lucky. After realizing that obstetrics was impaired by inadequate research and anachronistic care guidelines, I fought for diagnosis and got treatment the next time. My son was born on April 13, 2004: my fifth pregnancy, and the only one I've ever carried to full term.

After the six-year struggle to build my family was finally over, I still missed all the children I'd lost. I began to wonder why obstetricians had been so complacent with my miscarriages, and whether my children could have been saved if I had gotten better medical care. These questions continued to gnaw, so I sought answers by examining more than one hundred medical studies and interviewing researchers, physicians, and government administrators; I concluded that diagnostic care after loss is grossly inadequate, and women routinely lose babies that could have been saved if the medical community were more vigilant about preventing pregnancy loss.

The first step to preventing unnecessary miscarriages is for women to request a basic test—fetal chromosome analysis—after any suspicious pregnancy loss, meaning any second or subsequent pregnancy loss, any first loss that developed beyond six weeks gestation, and any loss when the pregnancy relied on assisted reproductive technology, such as in vitro fertilization. With this basic test, we could separate women into two groups: Those who have likely suffered bad luck, and those who require further testing to protect future pregnancies. But instead of a basic diagnostic test, doctors offer women unconfirmed speculation about how miscarriage "just happens," and that they simply need to "try again"—as if pregnancy is no more significant than the swing of a bat. This counsel implies that the life just lost had no inherent value, and that if women continue to try and eventually succeed, all their past losses will not matter.

But lost babies do matter; our children are not interchangeable.

To Full Term is the true story of my struggle to have a family, a memoir that begins when I discover I'm pregnant for the fifth time. I share this story to illustrate the devastation that still lingers after miscarriage, the anxiety of pregnancy that follows loss, and the strain that loss places on marriage, but mostly to show my readers why they must demand diagnostic testing after pregnancy loss.

My story illustrates what's at stake when women do not get adequate testing after miscarriage. And by sharing my story, I hope to save families and their unborn children from the devastation of preventable loss. I've woven findings from key medical studies throughout the narrative. Each study is cited at the end of the book in case readers want a deeper look at any of the research, but my goal is not to transform my readers into experts on causes of miscarriage; it's simply to persuade you to demand diagnostic testing after pregnancy loss and to spare you the horror of losing children that could have been saved.

I have included a section at the back of this book titled "What Every Woman Should Know About Pregnancy Loss." These pages outline some of the major issues in obstetrics, allowing the reader to make an informed choice about whether she needs to get more involved with her care. You'll note that many critical questions lack definite answers, offering only schools of thought because adequate research that could shed a clear light has not yet been funded. In past decades there were few treatments to prevent pregnancy loss. Dedicated researchers have miraculously worked with scant dollars to develop effective treatments, but to create benefit from these advances, physicians must begin viewing miscarriage as a legitimate medical condition that warrants preventive treatment.

The words you will read are true—all of this really happened to me. Although I changed the names and personal details of my medical professionals, after losing my twins in California I met several diagnostic physicians who were exceptional. And my two Boston-area physicians were competent and compassionate. They allowed me to participate in my care decisions, understood my anxiety, and never once made me feel like a bother with all my questions and concerns.

If you are reading this story and have experienced loss, I am sorry for your tragedy. I deeply understand the pain, the yearning for children lost. I encourage you to seek appropriate testing and the care of compassionate physicians who will deliver more than mere placations about how miscarriage is just "nature's way of taking care of a problem." If you get that speech after a suspicious loss, insist on testing or find another doctor who will administer the right diagnostics to protect future pregnancies.

Too many women are never offered testing after a suspicious loss, taking away their right to participate in decisions about their medical care. After reading this story, I hope more women will understand why they must demand diagnostic testing after a suspect miscarriage, and refuse to unnecessarily lose their next baby.

"It's time that physicians get serious about preventing miscarriage. When a baby is lost, it's a huge tragedy. These women deserve thorough testing to identify problems and prevent other losses."

> —Dr. Alan Beer, whose life's work was to help women with little hope build the families they longed for

"Physicians must stop guarding the past. Today we have the means to deliver better obstetric care than past generations, and the obligation to do so."

> —Dr. Jonathan Scher, Mount Sinai Medical Center, New York City

AUGUST

The plastic test stick has two lines.

I should be thrilled. I wanted this. I try to imagine holding a tiny baby in my arms. Awestruck. But my thoughts quickly turn to all those other sticks with two lines, all the thwarted promise. My stomach churns, and it's hard to breathe.

I stare at myself in the mirror above the sink, blond hair starting to gray, blue eyes tired, fair skin pasty. Am I ready for this? What if I lose another baby? I open the bathroom door. Jon waits, hazel eyes wide, lips parted. His breath sputters, still labored from a ten-mile run. "Okay." I nod. "Here we go."

With each passing pregnancy, I've told him with less and less fanfare. The first time, we were in a restaurant. The second time, I teased him on the phone about the secret I couldn't reveal. For the third, I left the test stick on the bathroom counter, asking him to bring me the sunscreen, the lotion, an endless list of urgent requests before he finally spied the stick. I can't recall how I told him about the fourth.

I remember every detail of telling him about the losses.

"Yes!" He presses me against his sweat-drenched shirt.

How can he still react this way? I step back toward the doorway, away from his blind enthusiasm and his smell. The test stick lies flat on the otherwise empty counter. I stare like it's a tarot card instead of a simple binary test. "How could this have happened right now? We stopped trying. I was using the ovulation predictors to know when not to have sex."

"When did we stop trying?"

"Remember? We were going to get settled?" I walk into the nearly empty bedroom of the new home bought just last week. "The moving truck hasn't even gotten here from California yet."

We stand amid bare eggshell walls with white sconces and windows without curtains. The renovated house we just bought in Boston, away from the strains of our life in San Francisco, was decorated so neutrally that no potential buyer would be dissuaded. With only a few pieces of rental furniture strewn about the soulless rooms, it feels bleak.

I think back to the last time we stood in a new home in a new place: San Francisco, eight years ago. Our lives were all about the possibility of newlyweds in a new city. I had just finished graduate school at the University of Chicago and Jon had just started a job in venture capital. We shared late dinners during long workweeks when we divulged every minute of our days, then we spent weekends exploring coastal towns where we whispered our dreams and imagined the children we would nurture. Our lives seemed almost impossibly idyllic.

But that was before all the tragedy.

"This isn't the time to get pregnant. We agreed."

He concedes that he must have forgotten our conversation. "But we're going to have a baby!"

His fearless joy makes my chest sink. I've already lost four babies. Doesn't he realize I could lose this one, too? And if I do, will it be my loss, or our loss?

Every tragedy has wedged a slightly wider gap between us. The first happened when our daughter, Maddie, was born twelve weeks premature. We watched her through different eyes as she fought in a neonatal intensive care unit for nearly two months before coming home. And then the losses came, when pieces of me shattered and he struggled to understand why. I've spent the last six years stumbling from pregnancy to pregnancy, filling the gaps with work as my grief mounted, grappling to reconnect the strands of marriage frayed after repeated loss was borne so differently.

I now stand before my husband of nine years, our experiences already diverging at the very start of this pregnancy.

"I haven't even seen the new doctor here." I shrug my shoulders.

"Don't worry about the new doctor. Dr. Conover recommended him," he says, referring to my trusted specialist in San Francisco. "And he's at a Harvard teaching hospital. You know the guy's going to be great."

"I'm not scheduled to see him until late September. That was his first available." I called for an appointment in July as part of my master plan: Move to Boston in August, adjust Maddie to kindergarten, prepare for a pregnancy in the winter, or maybe the spring.

But this is only August. The moving truck isn't even here. Maddie hasn't started kindergarten, much less adjusted. And the last part of the plan isn't supposed to happen for months.

"So call him now."

I look at my watch. Five-fifteen. Damn. I need to start medication for the clotting disorder right away. I wince, thinking about the daily self-injections that may help sustain this pregnancy. *May* help sustain.

After all the diagnostic tests, doctors still aren't certain why I've lost four babies. Some think the cause is Factor V Leiden, a recently discovered gene mutation that affects 6 percent of women. This usually dormant defect is believed to be activated by changes in gestational hormones, and is linked to abnormal blood clotting during pregnancy that can lead to fetal death.

I am one of ten million women in this country who carry this genetic error; I am also one of the lucky ones—at least I know I have this mutation. Because testing is so rare, few women know they are affected. For some, this lack of knowledge presents no problem; many women with Factor V Leiden have normal pregnancies. Others do not.

Heparin, the prescribed treatment, is considered unproven in traditional obstetric circles; medical guidelines do not yet recommend this treatment to prevent pregnancy loss.[2] Despite strong and growing evidence, there have been no large treatment trials to date, and thus heparin is not offered by many mainstream physicians, especially in the first trimester. Among doctors who do prescribe heparin, most wait until the twelfth week of pregnancy to begin medication. But Dr. Conover, my specialist in California, starts patients on heparin before twelve weeks, believing that this medication can prevent both early and later losses from Factor V Leiden. He convinced me that I should start this medication the moment I knew I was pregnant.

"I hope the new doctor agrees to give me the prescription."

"He'll prescribe the medicine. You'll persuade him," Jon says with complete confidence.

"Jon, you don't know that," I snap, feeling like he's dismissing my fears too easily, fears spawned from contentious doctor visits when I had to push for conclusions and prod at diagnoses—when he was out of town, or in a meeting; when he wasn't there.

Just last year I gave birth to twins at five months. The horror of losing these children was so tangible that we both quaked. When the shock dulled, I *insisted* on a wide range of tests—well beyond the few tests considered "standard"—to look for a cause of loss.

I saw four doctors, asking each why I'd lost my babies. None could answer with certainty. One believed it was a clear case of cervical incompetence, a premature weakening of the cervix believed to be the leading cause of second trimester loss. The next swore there was no basis for the last doctor's opinion. Another thought the likely cause was my Factor V Leiden mutation.

That's when I realized that medicine is about probability, not certainty. Doctors pursue treatments based on the *likelihood* that something will work, not the *certainty* that it will. This element of chance is especially pronounced in obstetrics, where research is grossly underfunded, leaving doctors to develop diagnoses based on opinions and outdated guidelines versus indisputable facts.

Jon locks his hands behind his neck. "Okay. If he doesn't give you the medicine, go to the emergency room. Hell, let's go right now."

"Jon, an ER doc isn't going to give me medication for something doctors aren't even required to treat." My shoulders tense with his last suggestion. He never saw the doctors, so he still doesn't understand how I had to fight for diagnosis—how the medical community fails more than *two million* women who miscarry every year by ascribing their losses to "unavoidable acts of nature" instead of confirming their suspicion with testing.

Medical guidelines instruct doctors not to test for causes of miscarriage until *two or more consecutive losses*.[3] This vague direction gives primary obstetricians wide discretion on whether women get any testing. High-risk obstetricians regularly see patients with multiple miscarriages—three, four, five, or more losses—who have never been offered even the most basic diagnostic test: chromosome analysis of the lost baby.

After my first loss, I heard the explanation routinely given to women after miscarriage: *"It was probably nature's way of taking care of a problem. Half of all miscarriages are caused by chromosomal abnormalities."* At the time, I didn't see the inherent flaw in this logic: The other half are *not* unavoidable acts of nature; the other half are symptoms that something is wrong.

More than 60 percent of women who lose a chromosomally normal pregnancy have an undiagnosed but treatable medical condition.[4] Most of these women remain undiagnosed because testing after miscarriage is so scarce. The result? A likely seven hundred thousand women lose pregnancies to treatable causes every year—and that's only in this country.[5] My twins, lost while I went undiagnosed and untreated, were a part of this tragic phenomenon just one year ago.

I slump down with my back against the laminate headboard of the rental bed. Jon follows and sits beside me. "Hey. It'll be okay this time," he says, stroking my arm. I take deep breaths and look toward my husband, try to touch the elation of this moment that he can still embrace.

This time could be different. We're in a new place, getting a new start, away from the scene of all that we've lost. I scan the pale walls and restored floors and try to imagine the possibilities.

"But there were so many conflicting opinions, and we still don't know if any of the doctors were right." I've pored over piles of medical studies, discovering research that could support every opinion I heard, then others that contradicted studies just read. After all the consultations in California, grasping for a degree of certainty that doesn't exist with subjective medical opinions, I had finally settled on a plan for the next pregnancy: Treat both of the diagnosed conditions because doctors can't be sure which caused my losses. This plan requires that I start heparin immediately.

"Dr. Conover wanted me to start heparin right away, but other doctors didn't agree."

"Look. It's going to be okay. I know you're worried, but it'll be different this time. We know what to do now. You have to believe." He gently squeezes my hand.

I stand and smooth out the Holiday Inn–looking quilt that came with the rental bed. "Appointment or not, I have to see the doctor tomorrow. Maybe I'll just show up at the office tomorrow. They'll have to do something with me. Wanna come?"

"I can't. My flight leaves at seven-fifteen. I'm in Raleigh, remember?"

I glance out the window and try to push aside my thoughts of another contentious doctor's appointment, again fought alone.

"We'll get it on my calendar for next time, okay?"

"Sure." I look at Jon, his face loving and sincere, and remember how the last tragedy changed us both, how this pregnancy will surely be different. He grabs both sides of my face and plants a sweat-covered kiss on my lips before starting to sing.

"We're gon-na have a ba-by. Gon-na have a ba-by. Buh-buh-buh-buh, buh BUH." He waves his hands while dancing a one-man conga down the empty hallway.

"We can't tell Maddie. Jon?" I stick my head around the corner to calm his thoughtless joy as his voice goes silent.

"Tell me what?" Maddie takes the last few steps up the staircase before stopping in the hallway. "What was Daddy singing about?" Her golden-red hair hangs in damp ringlets, and the freckles tossed across her fair cheeks look darker beneath her sunburn. I gaze at my only child, born three months premature, my living proof of a miracle.

"Nothing, baby. Did you have fun in the sprinklers with your new friend?"

"Is it a surprise? Do you have a surprise for me?" She squeals and leaps onto our bed.

"Yep." Boy, do I ever. I think about how she mothers all the younger kids at the park, and imagine her face filled with amazement at the sight of a new baby. Then I push aside this precarious image.

"What is it? Is it a dog? Are we going to get my dog you said I could have when we got to Boston?"

Who taught this kid to talk like a lawyer at five? "It is not a dog." The bribe-our-only-child-into-moving dog faded as the second line emerged on the pregnancy test. "But you're gonna like it."

"What? What?"

I smile, buying more time before falling back on her consistent favorite. "It's a really, really, special, yummy dessert."

"Yeah! Dessert!" She bounces in tall leaps. "Can I see it?"

"Not yet. Then it wouldn't be a surprise." I leave the bedroom and walk down the stairs, passing Jon at the bottom.

"Where are you going?" he asks.

"To that bakery we saw up on Lincoln Street. I am pregnant, you know."

AUGUST 26

My watch hits nine o'clock. I grab the cordless handset and dial, sitting on the floor surrounded by the essentials for my conversation: Palm Pilot, medical records, full cup of Starbucks. Maddie plays upstairs, watching the TV borrowed from the only friends we have in Boston. The office answers. I clear my throat.

"Good morning. I'm a new patient of Dr. Black's, and I'm pregnant. I need to see him today." The receptionist asks me to hold for the nurse who approves same-day appointments. I study my barren dining room and uncovered windows before Shirley comes on and introduces herself.

"I really need to see Dr. Black today. I'm a high-risk pregnancy, and I need to start medication immediately."

"Uh-huh. What was the date of your last cycle?"

"The date . . ." I open the memo titled "cycle" in my Palm Pilot, then scroll down the single column of dates that consist of a month and a number. Once the dates start to include the year as well, I know I'm close to the bottom. "July twenty-seventh."

"July. July twenty-seventh." Her voice trails off before going silent. "Okay. So you're four weeks pregnant?"

"Sounds right. I just took the test last night."

"And when are you scheduled to see Dr. Black?"

"September nineteenth. But I need to see him now. I have a blood clotting disorder. I tested positive for Factor V Leiden." I swallow.

"Uh-huh."

"I just moved here from California, and my doctor there, Dr. Conover, said I needed to start heparin the moment I knew I was pregnant." I'm up now, and start to pace with the closed Palm Pilot clutched in my hand. "That's my best shot at sustaining the pregnancy."

"So on September nineteenth, you'll be in your seventh week."

"Okay. Sounds right." Did she hear what I just said?

"Dr. Black usually doesn't see patients until their eighth week. But you haven't had your initial visit?"

"No, I haven't. But I need to come in today to start the heparin. I need a prescription today, and I need someone to show me how to inject it."

"I could see about getting you in a little earlier since you've never been in. Can you come in September the twelfth at two o'clock?"

"No. No. That's not good enough." I pace faster and shake my head. "Shirley, I really need to start heparin today. I can't wait nearly three weeks to come in."

"Miss, Dr. Black doesn't start patients on heparin until week twelve."

I stop. The line is silent except for the growing sound of my breath. "But I need to start now. Dr. Conover said I should start the medicine as soon as I was pregnant. Look, in California I was going to the hospital every month at day twenty-five of each cycle for a blood test. Every month. So I could start the medication the moment I was pregnant. We didn't even want to wait the extra three days for a pregnancy to show on a urine test. And you're telling me that I can't have the medication until week twelve?"

"What's your history?"

"I've had lots of losses." I throw my shaking hand up as though her question lingered in the air to be swatted. "I've lost four babies. Four babies. And my daughter was born at twenty-eight weeks. She's all right, didn't have any permanent disabilities, thank God."

"So you've had five pregnancies with one live birth?"

"Four pregnancies. I lost twins at twenty weeks. One year ago." I press my fist against my lips and breathe into it as if I could capture all my anguish and cast it away. "We're not sure if I lost them because of the clotting disorder, or because of the cervical incompetence."

I rush to justify the latter diagnosis, a premature weakening of the cervix, treated with a surgical cerclage. Medical guidelines say that doctors should consider this treatment when patients have a history of second- or third-trimester loss.[6] But how many losses constitute a "history"? Some cautious doctors believe only one, suggesting preventive treatment after a single late loss, while others offer no treatment until three or more late losses. Accepted medical procedure—women often endure three or more devastating losses before being offered care for cervical incompetence. I wonder how many losses Dr. Black considers a history?

"So I need to treat both conditions this time. I need to do everything I can, and I believe I should start the heparin now."

"You've had a hard time," she says after a long silence.

My shoulders drop and I bend to sit down again. "I'm very lucky to have my daughter. Shirley, I'm just so lucky. She's big and healthy. Tallest girl in her class. You'd never know she was a preemie."

"How old is she?"

"She'll be six in November."

"No developmental problems?"

"No. We were so lucky. And I really need to get this one through. I need to do everything I possibly can, you know?"

"Yes. I understand. But Dr. Black does not prescribe heparin until week twelve."

〜 AUGUST 27

I step through the open doorway into dim light, a welcome relief from the fluorescent glare of the hospital's hallways. The two purple tweed sofas and four matching chairs sit stiff and empty, as if unused. Faux wood tables house magazines precisely arranged as if painted on top instead of stacked. I walk toward a receptionist counter where an auburn-haired woman pecks firmly at a keyboard. I wait until she looks up. "I'm here to see Dr. Randolph."

She says her name is Lisa before exchanging my insurance card for a clipboard with new-patient forms. I unzip my oversized black tote to remove the folder with my medical records. It's about three inches thick, organized chronologically and held closed with two large rubber bands. "Here are my records from California."

"Great. I'll copy these."

"No need. That is your copy. And thanks again for working me in." After the dead end with Dr. Black's office yesterday, I called more than a dozen doctors before finding one who would see me today. "I cannot tell you how much I appreciate this. Thank you." I truly am appreciative, but I'm really here to get the heparin. I went from screening the supposedly best and brightest, away from the hospitals with international reputations, to the doctor at a local hospital who would see me immediately. I can't help but wonder: Why could he see me so soon?

I take the forms to the couch and sit on cushions that feel like cement. The first form asks for the CliffsNotes of my medical history. There is a grid on the top of page two that asks for dates and places of each miscarriage, stillbirth, and live birth. I hesitate before filling this out, not knowing how to categorize my twins. I bite my lower lip as I put them on the live birth line and note their gestational age, then hurry through the rest of the forms before handing them back.

"Hello. Darci?" A tall, fair-haired man in pale blue surgical scrubs stands with his hands resting on his hips, appraising me like a farmer assessing crops. "Dr. Randolph. Let's go back."

I grab my tote and follow him through a narrow hallway made smaller by unpacked boxes pushed against white walls. None of the usual baby collages or posters hang on the walls. They are bare. We go into a tiny room filled by a small round table and three chairs. Large lights embedded in the dropped white ceiling overwhelm the room with brightness, and as the doctor closes the door and wedges behind the table, I feel like a boxed lab rat.

"Have a seat, Darci."

I sit silently while the doctor turns the pages of my file. As he scans the call notes, hospital summaries, and test results, his face puckers with intense concentration. The quiet is occasionally disturbed by utterances of "uhm," and "right," which he seems to be directing toward himself. After several minutes, he pushes the file back and relaxes into his chair. "Okay. So you're pregnant. Congratulations."

"Thank you. It's a little surprising. My husband and I weren't exactly trying right now."

"Yes. Well, that's often how it happens," he says, rolling a wooden pencil between his fingers. "So let's talk about your history."

"Okay."

"You tested positive for Factor V Leiden?"

"Yes. That's why I want to start heparin today. My specialist in San Francisco said I should start the anticlotting medication right away."

"You've consulted him?" He puts the pencil down.

"Not recently. But last winter we agreed on a plan—how we'd treat the next pregnancy."

"Not many people give heparin this early for Factor V. It's usually started later. Week twelve," he says matter-of-factly.

"I know that's the norm." His comment brings some relief. At least he does believe in treating Factor V—many physicians don't even acknowledge this disorder. "But I'm told there's anecdotal evidence that suggests a benefit from earlier dosing."

"That's not supported by any scientific data."

I nod in agreement. Accepted obstetric guidelines don't require treatment for Factor V Leiden at any point in pregnancy, despite fourteen studies that found that women with inherited thrombophilias—the technical name for gene mutations that cause abnormal clotting—are more likely to suffer multiple losses.[7] "I know the science isn't perfect here. There are still a lot of unknowns."

Women with the Factor V mutation are thought twice as likely to suffer multiple early losses, and eight times as likely to know the horror of late losses.[8] In one treatment study, in which pregnant women with Factor V Leiden were given heparin, only 30 percent of these treated women miscarried; without treatment, 56 percent lost their pregnancies.[9] Despite this and other similar treatment studies, and despite the high prevalence of these mutations, obstetric guidelines still do not require doctors to test for inherited thrombophilias after recurrent pregnancy loss.

One of the strangest things about this disorder is that some women with Factor V have normal pregnancies while others develop clots that prove fatal to the baby. Scientists still don't understand why.

If only there were some way that this doctor could look at me, scratch my skin, read my palm, something that would reveal whether I'm one of the ones who will lose my pregnancy without the medication. But there's not. There are only odds.

"The thing I don't understand is why women aren't routinely tested for this, especially if there's a history of late loss in their family." Inherited thrombophilia means that the mutation was passed down across generations. Affected women often have mothers or sisters who have suffered late loss. My mother had several late losses. This should have raised suspicion about my condition, but few obstetricians gather a family obstetric history, never collecting these critical clues.

"We have the science to detect it, the medicine to treat it. So why are we letting women lose babies when treatment is available?" I find myself glaring at him as though he, personally, had something to do with the insufficiency of medical standards.

He takes my question as rhetorical, turns his attention toward my medical CliffsNotes, and picks his pencil back up.

"So, Dr. Randolph, is there a downside from starting the medication earlier? Is there any risk?"

"Well, it's never good to take any medication that isn't necessary."

"But is there a risk?" I know I'm pushing, and I study his reaction. He doesn't seem agitated as he contemplates his answer.

Dr. Randolph carefully reviews the possible risks, and then says the incidence is low. "The most common risk is from accidents. If you were to be in a severe accident and you were anticoagulated, you could bleed to death."

"But it's the same risk whether I take it sooner or later, right?"

"That's true."

"I want to treat it aggressively. If there's a chance earlier dosing may help . . ."

He doesn't respond. I sit back, run my fingertips over the tiny divots embedded in the table's edge. "Dr. Randolph, I still don't know for sure whether I lost my twins because of the clotting disorder or the cervical incompetence. I've heard different opinions about what caused my losses." We talk about the art in medicine, and how treatment is often subjective. As we speak, the sharp angles of his face remain relaxed, nondescript.

"Alrighty," he says. "Let's talk about your twins." He turns to the forms I'd completed earlier and scans. "You lost them last July."

I feel hesitant. He didn't say he'd give me the heparin. But my gut tells me to move on for now. "Yes. Thirteen months ago."

"Tell me about that."

I clasp the seat of my chair to steady the sensation that I'm sinking to the ground, the sensation that comes every time I think about them. "The pregnancy was difficult. It felt like everything that could possibly go wrong did. I had a lot of bleeding."

"When did the bleeding start?"

"Early. About six weeks."

"Do you know what caused it?"

"We're not really sure."

"That's not uncommon. The cause of bleeding often cannot be established."

I nod, having heard this many times before. "When it

started, it was heavy. Like something just burst. I went on bed rest for twelve weeks. Then my doctor said I should get up, that I was fine."

I press my fingers against my lips, trying to hold back my own relentless questions, the ones that still wake me at night. "I lost them two weeks after the doctor said I could get up. I think I might have kept them safe if I'd stayed on bed rest."

"Hard to know," Dr. Randolph says. "And were you taking heparin during the pregnancy?"

"No. I didn't know I needed it. I wasn't tested for clotting disorders until after I lost my twins. And nobody offered the test to me—even after all that. I learned about it from my own research, and I specifically asked for the test." I pull myself back in my seat, try to quell my agitation with a mainstream medical community that allowed me to lose four children and then made me do my own research before getting thorough testing.

"The doctor who delivered my twins said their placentas were a tangled mess of bloody clots. He said the placentas looked abnormal." I stare down at the greens and grays and blacks interwoven in the carpet, wondering what I might be doing today with my one-year-old twins if any of the doctors had given me a wider range of tests two years ago. "After I lost them, I fell apart for a while. But then I started searching for answers." I look back at Dr. Randolph. "I found Dr. Conover. He's in San Francisco. Do you know him?"

"I can't say that I do."

His response makes me a little anxious. I think Dr. Conover is like a rock star in the obstetric community. I scan the bare white walls, devoid of the usual framed degrees and accolades that infer status in the medical community. There's an open box on the floor with what looks like framed credentials, but I can't see what they are. "He runs a high-risk practice in San Francisco. Dr. Conover performs more cerclages than anyone else in the country. Or so the practice thinks. I understand nobody really tracks those statistics."

"No. There's no data on how many cerclages are done each year."

"So, Dr. Randolph, how many cerclages have you done?"

His face twitches. He leans back.

I realize he may have found this offensive, but I can't leave his office without asking the question. A cerclage is considered minor surgery, just a few stitches around the cervix, but a critical component to treat cervical incompetence. I need to make sure he's experienced with this procedure. "I mean, is it something you do a few times a year? Do you do ten? Twenty?"

"It varies. I've never really thought about how many. I've done quite a lot; did a lot at Johns Hopkins. I used to do them for most of the physicians there."

"When were you at Johns Hopkins?"

"I just left recently. I came here to start the maternal fetal medicine practice," he says, referring to the high-risk obstetric specialty. He pauses, then leans in a bit. "So, your Dr. Conover, does he do a MacDonald or a Shirodkar cerclage?"

"I don't know. I'm not sure."

"Well, what you want is the Shirodkar. I mean, anyone can do a MacDonald." He says this like we're sharing an inside joke. Then he leans in a bit closer and begins to sew in the air. "It's just a simple stitch, right around the cervix," he says. "But the Shirodkar, now the Shirodkar's more complicated. You weave it, like this, you see."

I lean in to watch his hands as he laces imaginary stitches with the imaginary needle held firm between his thumb and index finger. I've read about the two types of cerclages, but I really don't know the difference. "Uh-huh," I say, pretending to understand, wishing his fingers were leaving little jet streams in their wake.

"Now that Shirodkar's secure, placed high up on the cervix," he says with great pride. "That's what I do, the Shirodkar."

I study Dr. Randolph, this experienced, competent physician, as he beams at the thought of his beloved Shirodkar. From our meeting, I've tremendous appreciation for his patience, and my gut tells me that this man will give me solid care. "So let's talk about the game plan."

"Alrighty."

"I want to treat the cervical incompetence, and I want to treat the Factor V Leiden."

"Uh-huh."

"I want to do the cerclage. Dr. Conover said I needed it toward the end of the first trimester."

"That is when elective cerclages are usually performed."

"We also talked about bed rest." We discuss the use of bed rest in later pregnancy to help sustain a weak cervix, and measuring the length of the cervix to assess its deterioration during pregnancy. I tell him about my friend who needed complete bed rest to sustain the last ten weeks of her pregnancy—a necessity signaled by her diminishing cervix. "If they hadn't been measuring her cervix, they would never have known that she was at risk to deliver so early."

I look toward my medical records that lie open on the table, now disheveled, and wonder whether I can quickly find the copied pages of Dr. Conover's book about bed rest and cervical measurements. "I know a lot of people don't believe there's value in cervical measurements, and even fewer think there's any benefit from bed rest. But I do. And I think I should do it."

"There is evidence that supports bed rest during the later stages of pregnancy with a cerclage."

I exhale when he says this.

"But I don't believe there's much meaning in measuring the cervix." He says that the cervix is dynamic during pregnancy, and there are conflicting studies about the value of taking cervical measurements. "I do sometimes take these measurements, but cervical length varies from woman to woman, so the measurements don't have much meaning."

"But isn't the change important? If we're measuring my cervix and see unexpected changes, doesn't that tell us something?"

From his reaction he seems to be sizing me up. I feel out of place, arguing with a doctor over treatment options, but I need to do everything possible to sustain this pregnancy. I don't know if I can bear the tragedy of another loss, or the guilt from wondering if I could have done anything more. How can I not push for cervical measurements when Dr. Conover thought they were essential—the canary in the coal mine for his practice? "Dr. Randolph, I feel the measurements are vitally important." I stammer a moment, shaking my head.

"When I lost my twins, something wasn't right. I felt it. My old doctor, the one before Dr. Conover, met me at the emergency room. He examined me, said nothing was wrong. Then he sent me home. But he didn't do an ultrasound to measure the inside of the cervix."

I hear my voice shake, and I grip the arms of the chair. "I was back there, the same emergency room, twelve hours later. And there was nothing they could do." I look down, weighted with the culpability of demands not made, crushed by the longing for children I'll never know. "We might have known. If the doctor had done an ultrasound, if he'd measured my cervix, if I'd only insisted, we might have known . . ."

He watches, silently, his lips held tight. I place my folded hands on the table and take a deep breath before I lean in closer. My words are soft. "Dr. Randolph, I need you to take the measurements. Even if you don't believe in them, will you do it?"

He nods. "We can do it. I'll take the measurements."

"And we'll do the cerclage."

"Yes. Around week twelve."

"And I need the heparin. I want to start heparin today."

"All right. I'll send you down to the nurse. She'll show you how to do the injections."

A deep sigh rushes up from the pit of my stomach. He reaches across the table and gives my hand a quick pat before rising to leave.

SEPTEMBER

SEPTEMBER 1 *Five weeks*

"Taking a break?" Jon asks.

"Come join me." He closes the front door and slouches into the other cushioned chair on the wide front porch. After days of unpacking whenever we can, we still stare at boxes in every room. "Two boxes in the kitchen belong in our bedroom. Can you carry them up for me?"

"Sure." He rises from the wrought-iron chair. "Show me which ones."

"Not right this minute. Sit."

Since the pregnancy test, Jon has been admonishing me for lifting, careful to praise how much I'm getting done. I feel relieved from the contrast with the first few pregnancies, when he complained if I didn't feel well enough to go out; when he said I shouldn't succumb to my pregnancies. Then there were the early miscarriages—children I'd already held in my mind, lost before Jon had ever envisioned them. I still remember his confusion when my tears still came after months had passed. The twins were the first tragedy so tangible that we both felt ripped apart; Jon's understanding and acceptance are bittersweet, having grown after years of acrid practice.

"Cookie?" I ask, holding up the latest plate of homemade treats.

"Who brought these?" He scans the plate and takes the biggest one.

"The Schneiders. Three doors down." I toss my head to the left. "They have three kids," I say between bites.

"Three kids?" We discuss the dozen or so neighbors who've rung our bell, nearly all with three or four kids.

Jon reaches for another cookie. "You know, I don't want to sound unappreciative or anything"—he pauses while staring at the cookie, rotating his wrist, examining it from all angles—"but this seems so strange to me."

"What? The cookie?"

"No, not the cookie. That someone brought us cookies. That all these people are just coming right over, bringing us things."

"Jon, what's so strange about that? It's a friendly neighborhood. People just want to meet the new neighbors."

"I realize that. And it's great. Really. But it just feels . . . odd."

I laugh at my husband, still a cynical urbanite, uncomfortable with the kindness of strangers.

The air smells of freshly cut grass. Lawn mowers grumble in the distance. A light breeze floats over the porch as we watch an older couple preen their lawn, the husband plucking errant blades of grass as his wife kneels in a flower bed.

"You know what I've noticed?" Jon says. "Most people here cut their own lawns. I see people out with a mower, raking their own clippings. I haven't seen a single landscaping service yet."

We both look to our own side yard, the small swatch of land struggling under the shadows of towering conifers. Sparse blades of grass struggle to grow under the cover of pine needles. Jon stands and walks to the edge of the porch, hands on his hips, studying the challenge. "I should throw down some seed. Maybe in the spring," he says. "We'll have a full lawn next year."

I'm relieved as he stares starry-eyed at our barren plot of suburban dirt. I've worried that he won't like our new life here. He can't run outdoors year-round, and he's no longer in the epicenter of his beloved technology industry. I smile as he surveys our unfruitful earth, then turns to me with a huge grin. "Know what else?" he says. "When we get the grass, I'll mow it. Myself."

I laugh out loud at his excitement over lawn chores. "It's time to get Maddie. I'm off."

"Whose house is she at again?"

"Thaxtons'. They brought over bread earlier today and asked Maddie over."

"And how many kids do they have?"

"Four," I shout back, halfway across the street.

SEPTEMBER 4 *Six weeks*

"My girls like simple stuff. Chicken with broccoli. And maybe rice. Does that work for Maddie?" Mary hands me the Chinese take-out menu.

I stand in my new friend's kitchen where art projects paper the walls and scan the menu. Mmm . . . General Tso's chicken . . . fried chunks of chicken, somehow still crunchy in the tangy, sweet sauce. I order the chicken and egg rolls for myself. I'd also like the vegetable dumplings and scallion pancakes, but resist the hormones that urge me to binge. I look at Mary, thin, blond, dressing up a T-shirt and jeans with a bohemian scarf even while piddling around the house. So fashionable, her pajamas are probably even stylish. Pajamas? No. She seems like more of a long silk gown type.

My current lack of style is exceptionally apparent next to Mary. I used to be stylish, pairing fashionable suits with funky jewelry, sporting trendy hairstyles, and always in heels. That's all changed these past six years, a continuous cycle of gaining weight during pregnancy, then trying to lose the pounds after each loss. I'm too practical to buy new clothes when another pregnancy seemed just around the corner, and at some point, I lost the energy to worry about my hair. I stand here today, crumpled T-shirt hanging over my fat jeans and scuffed Keds kicked off by Mary's door, wondering whether I even remember how to be stylish, and hoping this woman isn't simply too chic to be my friend.

"I remember meeting you at Steve's wedding," she says, referring to our common friend. "You were wearing a blue dress, and I remember your hair being really blond."

"You have an amazing memory." That was eight years ago, the only other time I'd met Mary. I have no idea what I wore to Steve's wedding. But her second comment proves that I really must start doing something about my graying hair. I offer to help set the table and she hands me only five plates. I ask if her husband is joining us.

"No. He's in London, for work. He gets home tonight."

"Jon's been gone this week, too." I prefer when he's home, but I'm hoping he front-loads his travel into the start of the pregnancy, before things get harder. "He gets home late tonight, just in time for the big day. Can you believe our daughters start kindergarten tomorrow?"

We call the girls to dinner as the food arrives. I reach for the bags and my stomach curdles. Garlic chicken and boiled greens vent upward. Color fades from my face. Good grief, what if I throw up in this woman's kitchen?

"Are you all right?"

I don't know what to say. I can't tell her about the pregnancy. What if I have to tell her about my loss the next time we meet? My first two miscarriages were early, before anyone could tell. But I was five months pregnant when I miscarried my twins. Everyone knew. And I still sting from how some people treated me after losing them. Two moms from Maddie's preschool saw me at the library, just after my tragedy. The moms stared, eyes bulging, mouths open, as though my loss were contagious.

"I'm okay. But can I use your bathroom?"

I splash cold water on my face then sit on the floor. Thankfully, the nausea comes only with strong smells. I wait and join the group at the dining room table, surrounding my space with cartons of white rice and plain chicken skewers, hoping my behavior doesn't seem odd to my new friend.

Mary fills my water glass before jumping right into conversation. "What made you and Jon move to Boston?"

"The schools. We decided to move because Maddie was starting kindergarten." When Jon and I toured our school options, when he saw firsthand the reality of California public schools, where quality somehow declines amid soaring real estate, he was finally ready to leave. "We have no roots here, but with Jon in technology, we have to live in a city with a large tech base."

I don't tell her the rest, how I had wanted to leave San Francisco for years, how Jon and I fought over the move, how that city became nothing more than a scene of loss for me.

"I understand you're a writer. What do you write?" I ask Mary, changing the subject.

"Travel articles. I'm a freelancer," she says.

"What a great job—going to exotic places, searching out the best of everything."

"That's how it used to be. Now I write about places I don't need to visit." She reaches over to cut Grace's chicken. "Are you working?"

"Not right now." I smooth the edges of the linen place mat. I've worked since I was sixteen, full-time through undergrad, paying my own way. As part of the move, I'm leaving my marketing career with pressured deadlines and late nights that thwart my ideal of motherhood, but I'm not exactly sure what I'll do. Other than Maddie's birth, I've always worked, and often felt largely defined by my work. Without my job I already feel adrift, sometimes taking my old employee badge from my jewelry box and staring at the familiar woman in the photo. "I'll think about that after we get settled."

We clear the dinner dishes and move to the living room while the girls play. When we get there, I don't know where to sit. Every corner of the vast room is inviting and beautifully decorated—something I could never say about my own home. I've no skill to decorate myself, and I'm too economical to pay someone else to do it.

I decide on the scarlet chaise with the silk pillows. After a few minutes, Grace comes in with a request that takes Mary away. I take the chance to unbutton the top of my fat jeans and make sure my baggy shirt provides adequate coverage. Mary returns, this perfect woman in this perfect house, and I wonder whether she'd ever mesh with my disheveled life.

SEPTEMBER 8

I stand wrapped in a plush white towel and consider getting back in the bathtub for a longer soak. After a moment of procrastination, I turn toward the medicine cabinet. Nine o'clock— time for the heparin injection.

After two weeks of daily self-injection the thought still makes me queasy. *But the needle's not that big,* I rationalize, opening the top of the alcohol bottle. The sterile smell stings my nose. I open the glass jar where cotton pads are stuffed so tight they burst from the container. *This is for my baby.* From the medicine cabinet I grab a prefilled syringe, safe in a plastic and foil package.

I hate shots. I've passed out while getting shots in doctors' offices. Twice. And now, each and every day of this pregnancy, I have to plunge a little blade of steel into my own flesh. This is my best chance to prevent blood clots known to develop with Factor V Leiden, clots that could mangle my baby's placenta or block my baby's umbilical cord. But will this work?

Without large clinical trials, the gold standard of medical research, some physicians remain skeptical about the efficacy of heparin as a treatment for Factor V Leiden. But several smaller studies have been done, each showing a benefit from treatment. In one particularly compelling study, a group of women had never had a single live birth through eighty-two collective pregnancies; with treatment, more than 80 percent gave birth to their first child.[10]

American College of Obstetricians and Gynecologists (ACOG) guidelines, the accepted norms for obstetric care, say that scientific proof is not yet rigorous enough to recommend treatment for inherited thrombophilias like Factor V Leiden. A randomized, control-placebo trial would meet their requirement for proof, but how feasible is it to complete such a trial?

The study would require that a group of pregnant women who have all suffered multiple losses be separated into two groups: one group that gets medication, and the other, the placebo group, that gets no treatment. Randomized means that women do not get to pick which group they enter—researchers do that. Who's going to sign up for that trial? What woman would walk away from protection against a disorder suspected of stealing life from her body? And given the growing evidence that thrombophilias causes recurrent pregnancy loss, is it ethical to ask any woman to do so?

The words of one noted specialist still ring in my ear: *"If doctors wait years for the clinical trials to happen, a whole generation of women may lose their chance at motherhood."*[11]

I bend the corner tab of the plastic package and pull the screeching foil from the adhesive before dropping my towel. After two weeks of injections, my hips are sore and purple like rotting fruit. I search for an unmarked spot within the rounds of bruises that bleed into each other before wetting the cotton pad with alcohol. My hips look hopeless, so I look over my shoulder, toward my backside. The rounded skin glistens after the soaked pad glides across. I take the needle and pull off the orange cap with a snap, revealing the silver spear, about two inches long. I exhale and wonder if I can focus on something to avoid the tenseness and hesitation that makes me pull back the needle before it strikes. Should I watch the needle driving toward my body, or focus on the skin, dimpling slightly before the point bursts through?

Despite all the studies, I still have some doubt about these injections. Not all pregnancies are lost when this mutation is present. Affected women can have one normal pregnancy, only to lose the next one. Researchers still don't understand exactly how the mutation impairs clotting, or why it does so only sporadically. Because no doctor knows which type of pregnancy this is—one lost without medication, or spared by the irregular disorder—I chose to treat the condition. I wonder how many of the other ten million women with Factor V have lost pregnancies to this disorder, and how many would have chosen treatment, if only someone had given them a choice?

I raise the needle and plunge it swiftly into my skin. The wound stings. I push the plunger and medication creeps through my flesh, burning. I pull the needle out, holding a cotton pad against a drop of blood, grateful to have this chance.

SEPTEMBER 9

"Where's Maddie?" Jon's eyes dart across the playground.

We look through the hordes of children who cover the school lot. I turn to the monkey bars where she was a few minutes ago. She's not there. I study the playground more intently. It's just past sunset, and with the light diminishing, it seems less safe. Then I see the white polka dots on her pink dress flash across the blacktop. "I see her. Over there. In front of the pizza table." Maddie races across the playground with a pack of girls. She lets out a shrill laugh, piercing through the noise of the other forty families at the kindergarten picnic.

"Can you believe this, Jon? We're just letting her go off on her own." It took me so long to be even a few feet away from her. I let her go in baby steps, waiting at the bottom of the slide while she climbed up, then standing at the edges of the playground equipment. Finally I made it to a bench. Despite the physical distance, my eyes never left her. I wonder if I would have been less vigilant without the trauma of her seven weeks in an NICU?

I can still see her, twelve weeks premature and barely three pounds, tubes down her throat, lying idle in an incubator as monitors measured her every breath. Jon used to say that she was a healthy baby who simply had to live in the hospital; I was tortured by the image carried in my head for most of her first year.

"Do you realize this is the first time we've ever done this? She's running wild in a sea of kids. We're not exactly sure where she is at any given moment."

"It's a kindergarten picnic. She's safe," he says, as though this had happened before.

"Was she any less safe at the playgrounds in California?"

He chuckles and puffs his chest out. "I didn't do that. See, that's your problem. Daddy lets her play."

"Oh, really? Then maybe you can explain that panic in your voice when you just asked where she was."

He smirks at me but doesn't answer. We spot a cluster of parents from Maddie's class and walk over. As we approach, another mom comes carrying a tiny bundle.

"I can't believe you made it," someone calls out to the woman cradling the new baby. A little round face with closed eyelids and gently parted lips is wedged between a blue knit hat and a fluffy white blanket. As the mother recites tales of sleepless nights and jealous siblings, I am overcome with tension. I haven't been this close to a newborn since I discovered my pregnancy. I inch closer to Jon. Our arms touch and he reaches for my hand, squeezing tightly. His face is blank, his body as stiff as mine.

The mother introduces herself to Jon, saying her older son is in kindergarten with Maddie. "Maddie is so sweet," she says. "When I dropped off David this morning, she ran over and patted Ryan's feet through his blanket. She seems so caring."

I nod politely while trying to push aside the memory of Maddie's wail when we told her the twins were gone. Her cries were weighted with more sorrow and agony than I thought possible for a four-year-old. The child psychologist said she had to grieve, just like an adult, and that she would move on with time. And she has. She no longer asks every day why the twins died, just every few weeks. I look around, finding her back at the soccer field. She stands outside a pack of boys who now scuffle in the grass.

Moms begin to march toward the playing field, wielding admonishments at their sons. The new mom calmly takes in the skirmish before motioning toward the field. "I should get him," she says. "Do you want to hold Ryan for a sec?" She stretches out her arms, passing me the baby.

My arms reach with an automatic response. I take the baby. The blanket is soft and plush on my fingertips, and as I fold him into my arms, I feel his warmth beneath the blanket. I stand there, holding this coveted little miracle, and bring him closer to me. He smells of Johnson's soap, and my shoulders start to melt as I inhale the once-familiar smell. Jon stands beside me, and we both stare, silently, at this perfect little face. His skin is smooth, his face round. He's still asleep, and his tiny pink lips open ever so slightly with the force of each breath. I lean my head closer to him, so my ear can pick up the little wisps over the chattering voices and clamoring feet, and I close my eyes to push aside all the rest.

"Those boys," the mother says. I open my eyes and pull my head up. "Is he still sleeping?" she asks.

"Oh, yes. Sound asleep. And he smells so wonderful. I'd almost forgotten that baby smell." I don't take my eyes off him while I gently place him back in the mother's arms. I feel calmer, contented. "Thank you," I say, meaning it more than she'll ever know.

~ ~ ~

I grope to find a light switch in the pitch-black living room as Jon closes the front door. "Okay, Miss girl. We stayed so long at the picnic that it's past your bedtime. It's a quick bath, then off to bed with you." Maddie nods and hurries up the stairs.

"Can you get her bath? I still have work to do," Jon says.

"Sure." I follow Maddie to my bathroom and start the water while she gets undressed. "You looked like you had fun tonight."

"Yeah. And you know how many cupcakes I had?"

"No. How many?"

"Four," she says, with streaks of blue icing still smeared on her chin.

"Wow. You scored." Maddie steps into the warm bath. She sits down and I wet a washcloth, squeezing the warm water atop her shoulders. Water trickles down her creamy little back in tiny shimmering streams. She sits, still, silent. I squeeze the washcloth again and again, until her eyelids look heavy, and her shoulders slump, and her head starts to droop. I gaze at this miraculous child, my child, and I realize that much of my earlier tension has melted away.

"Did you have fun at the picnic, Mom?" Her voice is soft and sleepy.

"I had a great time. There are so many nice mommies." We finish her bath, and she stands outside the tub, wrapped in a towel. Her wet hair hangs to her shoulders, and I begin to stroke it dry with a small towel. "Time for jammies, girl. And please pick out your clothes for tomorrow." She walks to her room, too tired for the usual requests to delay bedtime. I close the door behind her and start undressing for my own bath.

That's when I see the blood.

"Don't panic," I say aloud. I repeat the words in my head, but my chest heaves from the familiar threat of bright red blood, just like I saw when I lost my first baby at thirteen weeks, and later, with my twins. "Jon!" I yell out. Within seconds footsteps pound up the stairs. Jon bursts through the bathroom door.

"What! What!"

The room starts to swim. I sit and hang my head between my knees. "There's blood. Not a lot. But it's fresh."

"Go lie down. Come on." He hurries me into bed as though the whole thing will be moot if we can just get there in time. "What's the doctor's number?"

SEPTEMBER 10

Jon and I stare straight ahead in the empty waiting room. He slouches on the couch, legs extended, crossed at the ankles. I sit taut, like a paper doll made from thick stock. We hear muffled words through Dr. Randolph's closed door as he wades through an eternal phone call.

When we called the doctor last night, I knew what he would say: Lie down, come in tomorrow. I still had to call. I needed absolute certainty that my actions were right; that I was doing all I could. Reassurance is the only cushion against the ruthless second-guessing and piercing guilt when things go wrong.

"He seems responsive," I finally say. "We've never had a doctor return a call so fast."

Jon nods in agreement. I lean back and rest my head on his shoulder. When Dr. Randolph opens his door, we bounce up like we're spring-loaded.

He leads us down the vacant hallway with walls that are thankfully still bare. I can't help but remember the other walks I've taken under the same circumstances, where hundreds of baby pictures arranged in decorative collages made me long for what was inevitably already lost.

The doctor steps into a darkened exam room where recessed bulbs cast soft beams like little spotlights. One is directly over the narrow exam table, creating a glowing funnel surrounded by darkness, like a tiny stage. Jon takes a seat in the chair pushed to the corner, and as I undress he folds my clothes and places them on the stainless steel countertop. The papery disposable gown crinkles as I tie the waist with the plastic belt, then take my familiar place on the table, ready for inspection.

There's an immediate knock on the door. Dr. Randolph enters. "We'll do an ultrasound to try and locate the source of the bleeding." He grabs the transvaginal ultrasound—a narrow probe about a foot long that looks like a corded vibrator, but maybe for a horse. I smell latex as he fits a thin plastic sheath over the device.

The Sony monitor mounted high in the corner squeaks when he turns it down for my view. Lubricating jelly splats from a bottle. Then I hear a rhythmic huffing and zero in, following the sound toward Jon. His chest surges, as though he's just run for miles.

"Is it too early for a heartbeat?" I ask.

"Perhaps. You shouldn't worry if we don't see one today."

I nod and tighten my lips.

"Are you ready?"

I place my ankles in the stirrups and grasp the sides of the exam table as if I might fall off. He inserts the probe. It's cold. My muscles constrict. I take deep breaths, slowly exhaling. Images flash across the corner monitor. Dr. Randolph maneuvers the probe for the right view. It pinches with every movement. I bite my lip and focus on the screen's image—something that looks like a dark lima bean inside a cone of grainy light.

He inspects the screen with lips pursed, continuing to adjust the probe. I stop looking at the screen with unfamiliar images and watch the doctor's face. He stops to study the screen again, and then looks to me with a slack expression. "Okay. There's the sac."

"Is it intact?" I blurt out, remembering the frayed edges that signaled my first miscarriage.

"Yes, it is intact," he says.

I reach for Jon. He grasps my hand reflexively, never taking his eyes from the monitor.

"And this light spot," Dr. Randolph stretches to point toward a squiggle of light inside the dark lima bean, "that's the embryo." I study the screen, staring at the little squiggle, trying to look through the safety of clinical eyes while my lips part.

"Can you tell why I'm bleeding?"

He points to the screen where a small pool of blood is visible, explaining that it's likely the source of the bleeding. "It's very small. The size is reassuring. But given your history of bleeding and miscarriage, it is of some concern."

I'd like to ask what caused the bleeding, and when will it

stop, but I know there are likely no answers. So I look at the intact sac where the squiggle lies, and savor the proof; at this moment, I am not miscarrying.

The room is still until Dr. Randolph reaches over to adjust a knob at the bottom of the ultrasound controls. Tiny lines begin moving up and down on the bottom of the monitor, like a little seismograph. "There is a heartbeat," he says.

Jon drops his face into hands with splayed fingers.

There is a heartbeat. I watch the tiny lines roll their reassurance across the monitor before the lines freeze. I look toward Dr. Randolph, his lips pursed as he evaluates the tick marks.

"The heart rate is 112 beats per minute," the doctor says.

Something's not right. I remember the heartbeat we got with the twins at seven weeks. "Shouldn't that be higher?"

"We would like it to be higher," he says. "At this point, we like to see at least 125. That's the low end of the normal range."

"So this isn't normal?" Jon leans forward. "What does that mean?"

"It means we're in a gray area," he says, expressionless. "A heart rate below 100 usually means miscarriage. When it's between 100 and 125, we just don't know." His Adam's apple jumps as he swallows. "I have had patients who were here and went on to have healthy babies."

"What's the percentage?" Jon asks.

"I don't know."

"Are there any statistics? Is this stuff tracked?" Jon starts to raise his voice.

Dr. Randolph explains that there's little information about heart rates in the first trimester. "I can only say that we do occasionally see it. I have seen some positive outcomes."

Jon and I look at each other with eyes that see the implied

knowledge of the doctor's response. "What can we do?" I rise to my elbows.

"I'll have you back next week to check the heart rate. Until then, I want you to take it easy."

"Should I be on bed rest?"

"Not full bed rest. But I want you lying about on the couch. No housework. No cooking. No laundry. Nothing." He wraps up our questions and heads for the door.

My mind is numb. I am ravaged by the thought of losing another pregnancy, once again just this side of seeing the family I ache for disintegrate. I stare at the monitor, the image of my little lima bean still frozen on the screen. Then I look toward Jon, wondering if he feels as pillaged as me, whether he'll share my anguish or hold it distant.

I wipe my tears and start to dress before Jon buries me into his chest.

~ ~ ~

"What can I get you for lunch?" Jon's voice is soft, gently prying open the silence that descended after we left Dr. Randolph's office. I lie on our sofa where Jon stuffs pillows behind my back and pulls a blanket past my shoulders as he offers to go to the grocery.

"Before you go, can you look through the boxes of books in the basement? I need the one labeled 'pregnancy,' and my laptop, please."

Part of me wants to just sit and cry. Another part wants to call the women who'll cry with me: my mother-in-law, my sister, my friends who have shared the emptiness and helplessness of every loss. But what good will my tears do right now?

I grab my computer and start googling "low fetal heart rate," side-stepping my turmoil and connecting to the familiar role of researcher. In my marketing career I've constructed volumes of research; I've designed study methodologies, developed recruitment criteria, and dissected results, separating the reliable from the biased, turning raw information into insights that could solve real problems. This experience has proven crucial in my struggle to have children, providing the means to deconstruct the wealth of conflicting information, and allowing me to stand in my steady career woman's shoes when I could easily wilt.

"What did you find?" I'm startled by Jon's voice as he walks toward the kitchen with bags of groceries. I hadn't realized he'd even left.

"There's not much on low fetal heart rate in the first trimester." I shake my head, feeling cheated. I knew about the Factor V Leiden, the cervical incompetence. I had time to research, to prepare. But now there's this.

Jon hands me a turkey sandwich laced with crisp lettuce and ripe tomatoes. I eat while we discuss the scant information available. I've found no relevant research studies, and because most women don't have ultrasounds so early, there may be nothing beyond anecdotal experience.

"Damn." Jon pushes his plate back on the coffee table. "Can't we have an easy one? Just one easy pregnancy?"

"I didn't expect this to be easy. But you know what?" I take a deep breath. "I wasn't prepared for the fear." I feel almost embarrassed that I hadn't anticipated the most obvious risk of all: the gripping terror that I may lose another baby. "I spent so much time thinking about the tangible stuff: medication, cerclage, bed rest. But the fear . . ."

"I'm sorry." Jon drops his head. "I'm scared too, you know."

I offer my hand and he squeezes it. We peer through eyes that reveal our fears, somehow lessening my anxiety and diminishing my apprehension that another loss might become a wedge between us.

"And the bleeding. Who thought we'd have this problem again." He throws his hand toward his memory of the bleeding that signaled the beginning of the end for my twins. We were at a restaurant, running from the table without even paying the check when I returned from the bathroom. I was six weeks along, the exact same time as now.

I feel gutted by such an immediate parallel with my last pregnancy. I also remember the sudden burst of blood, the race to the hospital, the bed rest for twelve weeks that was supposed to prevent the last loss.

After twelve weeks of bed rest I was told to get up, that I was fine; I lost them only two weeks after my doctor told me I no longer needed bed rest. And now here I am again, six weeks pregnant and bleeding, once again being told to rest, a questionable course of action that has already proven ineffective once. I still wonder whether it could have worked; if I'd stayed down, if I hadn't gotten up until later, would I now be facing the welcomed challenges of mothering twin one-year-olds?

My husband clears my plate and returns with a warmed chocolate brownie, the melted chocolate oozing from the sides. I stroke his arm. "Thank you."

⟡ SEPTEMBER 16 *Seven weeks*

"Jon!" I yell, sitting up from the couch where I've stayed for nearly a week. Jon's voice floats down from the second-floor office, wrapping up a conference call. I fidget, trying not to look at the clock. It's Tuesday, when Maddie is dismissed at twelve-thirty and needs someone to pick her up in the middle of the workday. I wait before heavy footsteps trample down the stairs.

"Thanks, honey." Jon hisses an extended breath as he rushes out the door. It's been six days since we saw Dr. Randolph. I've watched while Jon cleans, shuttles, and cooks while struggling to get his job done. I worry about the difficulty of our situation. Jon is self-employed; each day he can't work is a day he earns no income. Every time I look at him, his brow seems more deeply furrowed.

I go through the mail until Maddie bursts through the front door. "How was school today, sweetheart?"

"Great. Wanna see what I made?"

"Oh, yes." Maddie unveils her artwork while Jon rummages in the kitchen to gather lunch. He emerges with two peanut butter and banana sandwiches.

"Looks delicious." I bite into the sandwich made from two end pieces of wheat bread. Jon grunts while trudging toward the stairs, carrying a bag of carrots. "When is your last call today, sweetie?"

"Five. I should be wrapped up before six."

"Remember the sitter starts tomorrow. We have help soon." When the only college student who responded to my campus ad came to interview yesterday, I hired her immediately. What a difference from the first sitter I ever found for Maddie, the one I hired after screening forty potential candidates.

"Who's getting me tomorrow?" Maddie eyes me.

I remind her of the girl with thick black hair and pink shoes who drew pictures with her yesterday, explaining that she'll be picking Maddie up from school.

"Until you're better?" Maddie's face is serious.

"For a while." I wonder myself: How long will I need others to care for my child? "Maddie, you know that Mommy just needs a little rest to feel better, right?"

"I know. But you've been resting. Are you feeling better?"

"Yes. I'm feeling much better. But the doctor says it's a good idea to keep resting." She contemplates my response while we eat. We haven't told Maddie about the pregnancy—we can't risk exposing her to another loss. But how long is our lie to her sustainable? And what if she's worried? How long can I stay on the couch before she starts to create explanations in her own mind, scary ones?

"I'm glad you're better," she says, smiling as she hands me a card pulled from her backpack. On the front of the folded piece of pink construction paper is a large red heart. Inside is a picture of the two of us, her with red crayon hair, me with yellow crayon hair. We both wear wide smiles. She holds a balloon. Her card reads "git wil."

"Thank you, baby. You've already made me feel better." I put down the card and settle in for five hours of entertaining Maddie from the couch.

SEPTEMBER 19 *Eight weeks*

My eyes squint from the direct light over the exam table. Jon sits in the chair at my head, gripping both arms like an amusement park ride. I am draped in paper, ankles burrowed into stainless steel stirrups. An ultrasound technician with long brown hair adjusts dials on the equipment. Then she prepares the probe. Lubricant splats before she slides it in.

I stare at the blank ultrasound monitor, the one that will soon see whether life still exists within my body. I was eight weeks along in my third pregnancy when a similar machine looked inside and found no life; no heartbeat, just a hopeless sac starting to tatter. I had no bleeding, my body not yet recognizing the loss. Strangely, I also had little emotional reaction beyond numbness. I had insisted on testing after the first miscarriage, and after a few evaluations, my doctor believed that nothing was wrong; my inner voice just never agreed. With my doubts and the trauma of Maddie's birth and a miscarriage, I never risked a bond with my third baby, never let myself fantasize about holding the child or seeing the baby emerge safely from my womb. I felt emotionally unable to face another loss, so I distanced myself from the hopes and possibilities of pregnancy, retreating to a safer place, albeit an emptier one.

My third baby was sent for chromosome analysis; testing confirmed abnormalities. The obstetric community thus considered the loss "explained." So after one preterm birth and two miscarriages, no further testing was ordered.

"We're ready for Dr. Randolph," she says, stretching to hold the transducer in place with one hand while banging on the wall with the other.

My thoughts of what may soon be revealed are distracted by the squeal of a chair in the next room. In seconds, the door to my exam room opens.

"How have you done since last week?" Dr. Randolph washes his hands.

"I'm still bleeding. It's still red." I stare at the views that soon flash across the monitor, thankful that we haven't told many people about this pregnancy.

A few days after the shock wore off from the pregnancy test, we told Jon's family, my sister, and our few closest friends—the people we knew would share excitement over our news, but also support us if this pregnancy ends in loss. I'll speak to them all later today, after this appointment. I wonder if I'll hear their cheers or their condolences.

"How heavy is the bleeding?"

"Light. Maybe like the last day of a period."

"She's been resting all week. I haven't let her do a thing since last Wednesday." Jon puffs up.

The tiny lines appear at the bottom of the monitor. I watch the bars. They race across the bottom box, leaving a trail of little tally marks. Dr. Randolph studies them as they repeat. His face is blank; intent. The lines stop.

"The heart rate is 147."

I melt. Our baby has a strong heart rate. For today, our baby isn't doomed. Jon squeezes my shoulder and looks as though he's just gotten away with something. The corners of Dr. Randolph's lips slightly turn.

"Let's see you next week to check on the bleeding and heart rate. In the meantime, I still want you to restrict activity." He looks to Jon. "Keep taking good care of her."

SEPTEMBER 29 *Nine weeks*

"The heart rate is 157. Looks good." Dr. Randolph watches the gray tick marks float across the screen.

"Great." I lie on the exam table, taking in the baby that still looks like a lima bean in the images, but a bigger one, with a strong heartbeat. I don't feel tired and the nausea has subsided, but at nine weeks gestation, I'm still bleeding. We don't know why. "Can we get a cervical measurement today?" We talked about taking these measurements during our first appointment, intended to detect any weakening in my cervix. So far, we haven't actually done it.

"It's too soon," Dr. Randolph says. "The number has no meaning yet."

I want to ask why, but decide not to press the issue. He agreed to take the measurements, and because a loss from cervical incompetence shouldn't happen before the second trimester, his answer seems plausible.

"Get dressed. We'll talk in the conference room." The doctor leaves.

Jon and I chuckle while I'm dressing. He hands me my navy sweats, now replacing the too-small fat jeans. We go to the conference room where Dr. Randolph waits with folded arms.

"I think we should take you off heparin for a bit."

Jon and I are silent.

"I'm worried about the bleeding. It's light, and that is reassuring. But we don't know the cause. And heparin is an anticoagulant. It may be impairing your body's ability to clot off the bleeding," he explains.

"But what about the Factor V Leiden? Isn't there a risk of abnormal clotting without the medication?" Jon looks flustered.

"Possibly. But right now, I'm more worried about the bleeding. That feels like a more imminent threat," Dr. Randolph says.

"The bleeding has lessened. It's really not much more than spotting now," I rationalize.

Dr. Randolph waits, raises his chin a bit. "I'm not suggesting that you discontinue the medication for the rest of the pregnancy. But I think you should stop for a few weeks, just to see if it helps stop the bleeding."

I fall back in my chair. After fighting to get this medication, now I have to stop taking it? What if clots develop? If they come, they'll be silent, creating no symptoms until it's too late. What if this baby perishes because of my choice to stop or continue this medication? What if I make the wrong choice?

I feel sick from all the risk, all the crossroads created from one undesirable choice meeting another, each charged with their own unique perils. First the bleeding, then the heart rate scare, and now we have to decide whether to pause the medication that may have saved my other babies?

I look toward Jon. His face is blank.

Dr. Randolph waits, silently.

I lower my head and reason through my choices. *This mutation doesn't cause miscarriage in every pregnancy. Maybe it won't in this pregnancy. Maybe it will be okay for just a few weeks.*

I catch Jon's attention and nod. He nods back.

"Okay." I look toward Dr. Randolph, steeling myself to trust his judgment, and a little relieved to share some culpability for my outcome.

OCTOBER

"Wanna play?" Maddie stands by my bed, her golden-red hair gathered in two ponytails, like an Irish setter. She holds her Pooh in Candy Land game.

"Sure. Climb in." This may be our hundredth game since Sunday. I've spent the past few days in bed rather than on the couch, doing everything possible to stop the bleeding that's still bright red, still threatening my pregnancy. There are no scientific studies that say resting helps reduce bleeding. But some doctors swear by the value of rest to stop bleeding. And when I'm up more, I bleed more. My body tells me this is the right thing to do.

"I'm Tigger," Maddie says, grabbing the orange plastic tiger from the game box.

"Ok. I'll be Eeyore again." Maddie takes the first spin, fortunately getting a high number. She's especially sensitive today, crying when we had no milk, then again when her drawing went awry. "I feel so great today," I chirp while moving to the next blue space.

"Are you still tired?"

"Not much at all. I feel rested, Maddie. Mommy's healthy."

Her blue eyes flash. "Can we go out for a donut?"

"Well, no. I do feel great, but the doctor said I should keep resting." I wonder if she suspects my pregnancy. We can't tell her yet. There's too much risk. But how long can we maintain our lie that I simply need rest? She leans in to spin, then moves to a green space. We play in silence for a few turns.

"Mom?"

"Yes, Miss girl."

"Why did the babies die?"

I study the card I've just drawn, stare at the board for a moment. "The babies came too early. They needed to stay in my tummy longer, to grow more. But they came early, so they died. It was very sad."

She nods and takes her turn. "But *why* did they die? Why did they come early?" Her eyes are wide and insistent, her face weighted with confusion.

How can I best answer her? What words are there to explain death to a five-year-old and leave her feeling secure in her world?

"Maddie, there was something wrong with Mommy's body— something that's only a problem when there's a baby in my tummy—and the doctor didn't know. If he had known, he would have given me medicine, and then it would have been okay."

"Why didn't he give you the medicine?"

"The doctor didn't know I needed it, sweetheart. None of us did. But now we know. So if there's ever a baby in my tummy, I'll take medicine. And then it will be okay." My fingers sink into the pile of knit blankets pulled higher over my bulging stomach and I wonder whether my words are laced with detectable fear. What if none of this helps? What if my body has already developed clots after three days without the heparin I can't take unless this damn bleeding stops?

"I win," she says, guiding Tigger safely into the picnic.

"I can't beat you, Maddie," I concede. "What do you say we watch a show until Tiffany's back from the grocery?" I was surprised earlier when Tiffany, our college babysitter, offered to pick up bread and milk. Since she started two weeks ago, she hasn't been overly helpful. While we wait for her to return, I pull Maddie close and bury my nose in her raspberry-scented hair.

We watch a *Rugrats*. Then an *Arthur*. After leaving ninety minutes ago to get bread and milk, Tiffany opens the front door. "Tiffany, did you find the store all right?" I shout toward the stairs.

"I found it," she says, walking into my bedroom seconds later. "But I wanted to make cookies with Maddie, and they were out of cookie mix. I went to another store."

"That was so nice of you." I feel grateful. Maddie and I usually bake together every week, something we both miss. Now I'm feeling guilty that I questioned her. "Thank you, Tiffany."

"Cookies!" My bed screeches as Maddie leaps off, no doubt going to find her apron.

~ ~ ~

My lips part as I linger at the edge of sleep, breathing air laced with chocolate and sugar. This is the first time cookies have been baked in this house. I float downstairs to lie on the couch the few minutes until Jon comes home. Cookie sheets clatter from the kitchen before the oven door smacks shut. I meander in, expecting to find Maddie aproned up, covered in flour. She sits on a stool, quiet, clean, surrounded by hundreds of baked cookies that cover the marble countertops. Unused rolls of refrigerated cookie dough lie on the counter beside Maddie.

My eyes tally what must be a year's worth of cookies. "Tiffany, you *really* made cookies!"

"Well. Yes. But they're not all for you." She pauses, flattening out the crisp white collar under her red cashmere vest. "It's my turn to bring dessert tonight. For our dorm."

Her desire to "bake with Maddie" now makes sense.

"How many girls are you feeding?"

"I'm not sure. Maybe forty or fifty."

Breakfast and lunch dishes are piled in the sink, now accompanied by every baking sheet we have—and she leaves in ten minutes. "Jon should be home soon. I'm going back upstairs." I grab a cookie on my way out, then go call Jon's cell to share Tiffany's latest folly.

"She would be a perfect niece. She's so outrageous," Jon says. "But this isn't the kind of person we can rely on for help right now."

"I agree. We'll have to find someone else." We don't need a college student. We need a babysitter, a cook, a housekeeper, a laundress, a chauffeur—people to do all the tasks that I usually do. But other than a parent, who's willing to do these jobs?

"So what's for dinner?" Jon asks.

"I have no idea." After weeks of precooked chickens and takeout, I would almost prefer not to eat. But I'm pregnant, and hungry. "Can you stop on the way home and grab wraps?"

"Again?"

"How about Whole Foods? Do you want to pick up a chicken?"

"No."

"Then pick something else. I don't care."

"What else is there?"

"I don't know, Jon. I've been housebound since we moved here." We bicker through our options and then decide to make oatmeal for the third time this week. I look toward my closet, where dirty laundry spills from the door. "Do you have work to do tonight?"

"A few hours' worth." He pauses. "Why do you ask?"

"Well, I know you've had a long day—"

"A twelve-hour day."

"I know. Very long." I pause. "But we need laundry. I'm sorry to ask you this, but you'll need to do some laundry when you get home. And pick up the kitchen."

"Damn it." Silence. "You have to find more help," he commands, as though I'm turning people away. "Tomorrow."

OCTOBER 3 *Ten weeks*

"You are over thirty-five. Based on age alone, your risk for Down syndrome is 1 in 145, and for any abnormality, 1 in 83," Dr. Randolph says. "Testing is recommended."

We sit in Dr. Randolph's conference room, the sterile walls and industrial fixtures now as familiar as my own home, discussing whether we'll do an amniocentesis. "I don't know if I can do an amnio again. The risk . . ."

"There is some risk. About one in every two hundred patients will miscarry after the procedure," the doctor states.

Jon and I both sit up. I knew this statistic, but now it feels closer, like saying it aloud invited it in. "And from your experience with loss caused by an amnio, how many days after the procedure before a miscarriage actually happens?"

"When there is a loss, it usually occurs rather quickly—within days of the test. Theoretically, a loss could occur up to two weeks after the procedure."

"And have you seen that, losses caused by an amnio, but not until two weeks after the procedure?"

My stomach churns, stirred by the memory of losing my twins two weeks after an amniocentesis. Every doctor said the amnio did not cause my loss since I had no cramping or bleeding after the procedure—symptoms that should have come if harm had occurred. The abnormal clots in their placentas indicated Factor V Leiden played a part, and we know my cervix isn't normal; these are far more likely culprits. But the question still lingers: did the amniocentesis somehow contribute to their loss?

"No. I can't say that I have," he says matter-of-factly.

"There are other options besides an amnio to determine fetal chromosome status." Dr. Randolph discusses CVS, chorionic villus sampling, in which tissue samples are taken from just outside the fetal sac to evaluate the baby's chromosomes. This procedure is thought to have even more risk than amniocentesis.

"With everything we're dealing with in this pregnancy, I need to know that this baby is okay." I shrug my shoulders. "But both procedures sound so scary. I'm still bleeding, and we know my cervix isn't stable. It just sounds risky, snipping tissue samples when things already feel so shaky."

"The CVS is out," Jon says definitively, then looks toward me for confirmation.

"There is another option. We could do integrated screening." Dr. Randolph explains the noninvasive program that combines an ultrasound and blood tests taken at different points in the pregnancy. "We combine the data and calculate the likelihood of an abnormality based on more than just age. You could get something that comes back 1 in 3,000. Or, it may come back 1 in 10."

"How reliable are the results?" Jon asks.

Dr. Randolph explains that screening identifies women with higher odds of a problem, whereas a diagnostic test like an amnio confirms the actual presence of a condition. "This is not as reliable as amniocentesis, but it can flag close to ninety percent of abnormalities."

Jon and I exchange reluctant glances. This seems like a good option—more insight without more risk.

"Testing is always a choice. You don't have to do anything," Dr. Randolph adds.

OCTOBER 6

"Jon!" I yell from my bed. I've called out three times in the past fifteen minutes. No response. My bleeding became heavier three days ago. It had ebbed and I was up more—then it returned, heavier, and bright red. There's no cramping yet, but that can come all too quickly.

I fear that I'm just this side of loss, if not from the bleeding, then from the clotting disorder. Without heparin, medication we can't use unless the bleeding stops, my baby is defenseless against Factor V Leiden. Jon and I agreed that I should stay in bed—it's our best chance to stop the bleeding. Then he decided to work from the office in the attic, away from the distractions of his regular home office. Namely, my voice.

I call his cell phone. Straight into voice mail. Damn. "JON!" I scream.

"WHAT?" he yells from above, then says something I can't make out before stomping down the stairs.

"Jon. I've been calling you," I snap.

"I didn't hear you."

"And where's my bell?" I push up onto my elbows and open the now-empty nightstand drawer, where my little silver school bell usually stays.

"I hate that bell," he says, through near-gritted teeth.

"Well, I don't like it either. But we agreed that I should stay in bed, and I need your help." I throw back the blankets and sit up. "How do you propose I get your attention?"

"Just call out."

"That's not working." We stare at each other, frustration mounting. "I need water. And I've been getting up too much today."

"Can't you just drink it from the bathroom sink?"

"No. It's not filtered. It tastes bad."

He turns and leaves. Drawers smack and dishes clatter from the kitchen downstairs. He returns with a silver carafe of ice water.

"Here." He puts the carafe on the nightstand. "I need to get back to work."

"Thank you," I say, calmer. "Jon, I realize that you're self-employed. If you don't work, we've no money. I get that. But I also need help. So how can we work this out?"

"Hire someone, Darci. I can't do all this. I *can't*."

"I've tried, Jon. Geez! It's like you think there's a line of people outside our door who want this kind of work. Don't you get that I haven't been able to find anyone yet?"

Jon shakes his head, his face still flushed with annoyance.

"So until I can get help, how do I get your attention when I need you?"

"Yell when you need something." He turns and leaves.

~ OCTOBER 11 *Eleven weeks*

"We'll call you when we get to Stacy's," Jon says, referring to my friend in Chicago who will watch Maddie while he runs the marathon there. He has one hand on the front door, then stops again. "Are you sure you have everything?"

He went to the store and picked up enough prepared food for a week, plus three DVDs. "You'll be back tomorrow night. I'll be fine," I say. "Have a good race."

He stops, puts down his suitcase. "Are you sure this is okay?"

"Jon, for the tenth time, I'll be fine. I want you to go." My bleeding isn't bright red anymore, now a reassuring brown. I'm still on restriction, but I feel more confident sitting up, or walking to get my own water. Besides, he could be home in a few hours if something happened. With months of training and the stress of working while caring for all of us, he desperately needs this release. I'm hoping that this excursion quells some of the tension that's festering between us.

"And you promised Maddie that you'd show her all our special places in Chicago."

Chicago is where Jon and I met. We lived in the same high-rise apartment building. I had moved to Chicago alone, knowing no one, excited to leave Ohio and add more adventure to my life. I heard about a party on the sixteenth floor, and as a woman with nothing to lose, I crashed the party. Turns out, it was Jon's party. I still remember his struck expression when we met, and how he later persuaded our doorman to give him my phone number.

"I'll be right here on the couch, watching movies and interviewing sitters. There are four people coming today alone."

I found someone to come for afternoons, but she has her own children in school, and isn't sure how long she can help us. I need to find more help before Jon explodes from all the pressure. "You'll come back having run another marathon, and I'll have found another sitter." I lie back on the couch, eased by the thought of another babysitter to relieve some of our stress.

"Dad! Let's go before we miss our plane," Maddie pleads, clutching the extended black handle of her Scooby-Doo Pullman.

They come for one last round of kisses before heading to Chicago.

OCTOBER 14

"Hello!" Mary's eyes still look surprised from our phone call yesterday, when I told her about my pregnancy. It felt so awkward, explaining that I'm on partial bed rest, alluding to my inadequacy, so exposed to someone I barely know. Now she stands at my door. I reach to take the two coffees and the paper bag bulging with pastries that hangs from her hand.

"No way," Mary says. "Go lie back down. I'll do this."

I go back to the couch and try to get comfortable. This feels so strange—inviting someone over while I recline on the sofa. But I've had no visitors since we moved here, and the isolation is starting to get to me. I need to either get used to this awkwardness or accept the loneliness.

"I wasn't sure what you liked." Mary holds out a plate filled with berry scones, chocolate croissants, and cinnamon rolls. "I figured this was safe."

"You're so generous. This is wonderful. Thank you." I grab half of a blueberry scone. She takes part of a cinnamon roll and then sits in the leather chair across from the couch. I spill the details about my pregnancy.

"So what happens now? Do you just hang out here for the rest of the pregnancy?" She glances at my bare walls and sparsely furnished rooms. I sense that the lack of decorating alone would be untenable for her stylish sensibilities.

"I don't know. I knew I'd need bed rest the third trimester, but not this—not yet. I'm hoping I can get up when the bleeding stops."

"How are you managing the day-to-day stuff, like Maddie, and groceries?"

"We're barely managing anything right now." Old newspapers are tossed by the fireplace, the coffee table is littered with half-full glasses and an empty pizza box, and Jon's running clothes from yesterday are strewn across the floor. "I found someone to help out a few mornings, and another sitter starts next week for afternoons. Until then it's on Jon's shoulders."

I feel guilty about the burden of all this on Jon, and helpless when I can only watch as he dredges through our onerous reality. I comment on how hard all this is for him nearly every day. He says he knows it's hard for me too, but sometimes this knowledge seems muted by his huffs and exasperations when I'm forced to ask for one more thing than he can possibly do.

"I'm going in the kitchen to warm my coffee. Can I take yours?" I nod and Mary places our coffees atop the closed pizza box, then piles dirty glasses on top.

"Oh, Mary, you don't have to do that."

"I'm going in there anyway. It's nothing." I watch, awkwardly, as she clears the mess from the table. She comes back with my coffee, warmed, and a glass of ice water. We talk about the treatments needed during my pregnancy.

"I'm having a cerclage in two weeks, for cervical incompetence."

"My mom had that," she says casually, reaching for a croissant. "She lost two pregnancies, and then the doctors did something to support her cervix. That's when she had me." I take her in for a minute, a living example of how this can turn out.

We talk about the cerclage surgery—a plastic band placed around the cervix and woven through with stitches that are pulled tight, like cinched purse strings. "Once the cerclage is in place, and the bleeding stops, I should be able to get up. I shouldn't need bed rest again until later in the pregnancy."

Jon bursts through the front door, leaving a trail of sweat beads across the wooden floor. He sees my guest as he heads toward the stairs. "Hi. You must be Mary," he says. "I'd shake your hand, but I'm pretty gross."

"He just ran a marathon last weekend," I brag, glancing at his glistening runner's calves. Since the marathon he has seemed calmer, a little less tense. Jon makes small talk about running before excusing himself to take a shower.

"Is he usually home during the day?" Mary asks.

I explain that he's now working from home, given our circumstances.

"I'm sure you need that right now," she says, then leans in closer, lowers her voice. "But doesn't it, well, drive you a little crazy, spending that much time together?"

I knew I loved this woman.

ᴥ OCTOBER 20 *Twelve weeks*

"Dr. McConaughey." He extends his hand toward the exam table where I sit. Until today, I've seen only Dr. Randolph, a specialist, during this pregnancy. I'm required to have a regular obstetrician for standard prenatal care, such as checking weight, monitoring blood pressure, watching for the typical complications of pregnancy. Specialists don't spend time on these important matters, which they consider routine.

I feign a smile and reach out my hand. With every new doctor comes a potential new battle, another challenge of my treatment plan. But there's less controversy about the basic care Dr. McConaughey will administer. Most of the conflicts arise from the aberrant problems, those treated by Dr. Randolph, not the standard fare to be managed by a primary obstetrician. While we shake, he studies me with unwavering green eyes. Dr. McConaughey is strikingly handsome, with a strong jaw and wavy brown hair. His first name could be Matthew.

"I am glad you're here, but why haven't I seen you earlier? You are twelve weeks along."

"I know I was supposed to be here weeks ago. But with the low heart rate, and the bleeding, I've needed to see Dr. Randolph for ultrasounds nearly every week." We review the findings from my most recent ultrasound, a diagnostic tool unavailable in many primary obstetricians' offices. The discussion turns to my history, already documented in an hour-long visit with an intake nurse. "My daughter was born twelve weeks premature, at twenty-eight weeks."

"When you were in California, nineteen ninety-seven," he says with my closed patient folder still clasped in his hand.

We discuss my labor with Maddie, how it began with radiating back pain. "Maddie's birth and each loss started with the same strange back pain. Then the cramping came."

"The first sign of labor is often back pain."

"It's never a normal, throbbing backache. The pain radiates—and I've only had this type of pain when I'm in labor or miscarrying. The first time the pain came with Maddie, I didn't go to the hospital for hours." My voice sounds pleading, still weighted from the guilt of my ignorance. I had no idea the pain was labor, so I kept working—until midnight on a Sunday. I had a presentation Monday morning to corporate VPs who could approve a bigger advertising budget for my business, something that, at the time, felt of paramount importance.

"I had no idea I was in labor. No clue what it was supposed to feel like." I stare at the green tweed carpet, crisply recalling every detail of Maddie's seven weeks in the NICU, her tiny three-pound body a pincushion for the tubes, needles, and monitors that fed her, medicated her, and measured her every breath. I can't remember whether my business ever got the extra advertising spend. "For the first forty-eight hours, the doctors wouldn't even give odds for her survival."

"I'm sure that was difficult." He steps closer and leans against the exam table.

I nod and fuss with the plastic tie holding my exam gown together. We review the two miscarriages, then the loss of my twins. I emphasize the details that support my treatment regiment. "Dr. McConaughey, I'm worried that I'm going to lose this pregnancy. If I can make it past the bleeding, past the cervical incompetence, the damn clotting disorder—if I get past all that, I'm still likely to have another preemie." I stiffen and sit straight up.

"We will take great care of you. If you have any problems, day or night, call." He pauses before patting my arm.

My shoulders droop as I ease into the comfort of his manner. Then I remember that I need more than routine care from Dr. McConaughey; I need him to take cervical measurements. The plan is to see both doctors once a month, each taking a measurement at every appointment. Dr. McConaughey hasn't heard the plan yet—or agreed.

"So, Dr. McConaughey, I'm worried about cervical incompetence, whether my cervix will hold for this pregnancy. Dr. Randolph agreed that we would take regular cervical measurements—to track changes in cervical length."

I study his reaction, knowing this is controversial, a practice not endorsed by standard obstetric guidelines until multiple late losses have occurred. More than a dozen studies link short cervical length and preterm delivery in at-risk patients—the shorter the cervix, the higher the risk of preterm delivery.[12] Yet obstetric guidelines are vague about the need to take these measurements after only one late loss, implying that the horror of late loss should be repeated before preventive care is administered.[13] With Maddie's preterm birth somehow not counting, I'm technically considered to have had only one late loss; standard guidelines would require me to lose the baby I'm now carrying before preventive care is considered justified.

"When do we start measuring my cervix?"

He opens my file and studies it for a moment, then looks at

me over the top of thin Italian glasses. "You're scheduled to see Dr. Randolph today?"

"In thirty minutes."

"Why don't you discuss it with him, during your visit."

I don't know how to respond. Dr. Randolph hasn't yet taken a single measurement. When are we supposed to start? My California doctor wanted measurements taken every two weeks, requiring both my specialist and primary obstetrician to participate, but he never said when we should begin. "I'll ask him today." I feel more comfortable pressing Dr. Randolph, and besides, I can ask him in just a few minutes.

~ ~ ~

As I enter Dr. Randolph's office, Jon sits on the waiting room couch, busily tapping the keys on his laptop. He couldn't come to the first appointment with Dr. McConaughey, but he made it to the four P.M. appointment with Dr. Randolph. The nurse calls my name before I reach him. "Just in time," he says, packing up before we walk toward the exam room. We discuss my visit with Dr. McConaughey while I undress.

"How often will you see him?" Jon asks.

"Once a month. I should have already seen him once or twice." That was before all the unexpected threats to my pregnancy. I'm now again positioned on the specialist's exam table, the sixth time in six weeks.

An ultrasound technician comes in to start the exam. She studies images on the monitor for several minutes before summoning Dr. Randolph with an effective pounding on the wall. When he enters, we discuss my visit with Dr. McConaughey.

"He said I should ask you about the cervical measurements. When do we start taking them?"

Dr. Randolph pauses and looks at the views on the monitor. "I usually don't take measurements until later, week fifteen or sixteen." He explains that until the uterus is fuller, it's hard to tell where the cervix begins, thus difficult to determine where to anchor the measurement. Some research suggests that doctors often take inaccurate measurements because they misjudge where the cervix actually begins. "But your cerclage is in two days. We could take our first one today."

"Let's do that." I relax into the table, relieved that I didn't have to fight this battle again. Dr. Randolph maneuvers the transducer. Reels of black-and-white images flash across the monitor. I fruitlessly study the screen, like hieroglyphics I can't decipher. Then the image freezes, like a photo instead of live video. Two tiny electronic Xs appear on the still image. He repeats the procedure, making a second set of Xs, drawing a dashed electronic line between the two end points.

"What's the measurement?" Jon squints toward the screen.

"It's . . . about . . . twenty-seven millimeters."

"What's normal at this point?" I ask.

"There's no single right number." Dr. Randolph talks about how cervical length varies among women, and that the cervix is dynamic, often changing throughout pregnancy. "But I would like to see a longer length. Your cervix does appear shortened."

I'm not sure what to think. "How bad?"

"Well, I'm not alarmed, but I have some concern."

A study from the *New England Journal of Medicine* found that average cervical length is 35 millimeters; any number below 25 millimeters is a warning sign, revealing a higher chance of preterm labor.[14] For doctors who take these measurements, most intervene when the cervix shortens below 25 millimeters.

"But that's why we're doing a cerclage in two days, to reinforce the cervix before it deteriorates," he says. "With this number, and your history, it's good that we're doing the cerclage."

"Will the cerclage fix it? Will it definitely take care of it?" Jon interrupts.

Dr. Randolph purses his lips. "It likely will. Most patients with a cerclage carry to full term." He explains that by putting the cerclage in early, before the cervix has greatly diminished, the procedure is more likely to be effective. The cervix may not continue to shorten, and if it does, the cerclage creates one final barrier to prevent the membranes from prolapsing into the birth canal, an event that leads to early delivery in most cases.

"We're getting you just in time to do a Shirodkar cerclage," he says, referring to the type of cerclage he believes superior to other methods. "The stitch will be high on the cervix, and should provide strong reinforcement."

His words are reassuring, but I still feel scared, defective.

"I want you on full bed rest now, Darci. You're to lie flat, all day. No sitting up. No getting up for anything except going to the bathroom." I smirk toward Jon, feeling vindicated with our choice to remain on restriction after the bleeding finally stopped last week. He asks if we have any questions before turning to leave. "Alrighty. I'll see you Wednesday when Dr. McConaughey does the cerclage."

"What? Dr. *McConaughey's* doing the cerclage?" I rise up on my elbows. Dr. Randolph looks surprised.

"As your primary obstetrician, he usually does the procedure. Hospital protocol."

I feel okay about Dr. McConaughey. But I trust Dr. Randolph, and I know he has deep experience with this surgery. He told me about performing cerclages for most of the physicians at

Johns Hopkins. "I'm not comfortable with that. I want you to do the cerclage."

He raises his chin, studies me for a moment.

"Dr. Randolph, I've been seeing you for nearly two months now. I just met Dr. McConaughey for the first time today. This makes me very uncomfortable. I . . . I . . . ."

"All right, Darci. If you prefer, I can do the procedure. Dr. McConaughey will still be there. Two surgeons are present with any surgical procedure."

"I'm fine with that. But you'll do the actual stitching?"

"Yes."

I sink back into the table, but my eyes remain wide and fixed on Dr. Randolph.

⟋⟍ OCTOBER 22

Jon and I wait in the presurgery room, a loading dock for surgical procedures. A dozen patients in flowered hospital gowns lie on steel gurneys with scratchy white sheets. There's little chatter, just the hushed words of doctors and nurses. Jon holds my clothes in a plastic bag that crinkles as he passes it from hand to hand, glancing toward his briefcase.

"How are we doing this morning?" Dr. Randolph opens the curtain and steps in. "The OR is a bit behind. About twenty minutes." As we make small talk, Dr. McConaughey comes in. He's wearing a finely tailored dark suit, red silk tie, and crisp white shirt. The contrast with all the surgical scrubs and white coats stands out.

"You look so handsome, Dr. McConaughey." *Good grief. Did I just say that? Did I just call my obstetrician handsome?* My little curtained fortress is still and silent for a moment. Jon looks at me as though I just swore that Bill Clinton's picture is on the dollar bill. Dr. Randolph sways a bit, smiling, the first smile I've ever seen on his usually inscrutable face, making eye contact with Dr. McConaughey.

"I just came from a department meeting. But thank you," he generously adds. He asks whether I've signed consent forms, and confirms that possible risks from the procedure were reviewed: infection, contractions, miscarriage.

"So the likelihood of miscarriage after cerclage is low, maybe two percent? Is that right?" I ask.

"It's low. You may have a little spotting after the procedure. That's normal. But we want to see you if there's pain, cramping, or abnormal bleeding," Dr. McConaughey says. "You also need to call about any abnormal discharge. Infection is a risk." He pauses, keeps eye contact, his face calm. "We will take good care of you."

~ ~ ~

"Roll over on your side," the anesthesiologist says. "This will hurt for a minute when I stick you."

I gasp as the spinal is inserted. The needle is thick and long, a channel to funnel drugs through my spinal canal. The anesthesiologist had numbed the injection site with a local anesthetic before inserting the spinal catheter. But this needle is thicker, goes much deeper. After a few gulps, the pain subsides. I am awake, fully alert, but soon feel nothing below my chest. I cannot move my legs. Nurses and doctors tug at me, a sack of dead weight, pulling me from the gurney onto the stainless steel table. A young man in pale scrubs, maybe a resident, pulls the hospital gown above my hips, then steps back. His face contorts as though he's just seen some abomination, and with wide eyes, he whispers something to Dr. Randolph.

Dr. Randolph steps closer to me and inspects my midsection before turning to the young man with big eyes. "It's from the injections. You will see this sort of bruising with most patients on heparin."

I remember the posters taped to hospital walls imploring doctors and patients to report any sign of domestic abuse. The resident's face still looks disturbed when he's blocked from view by a papery blue tent draped above my chest, hiding the doctors who now gather at my legs.

"Let's get her into stirrups."

My legs are lifted, secured. I look around at the room, rather sparse except for the table where I lie, the five people scattered around the table, and the cluster of bright lights now directed toward my legs.

Dr. Randolph appears near my head. "We will take a quick ultrasound of the cervix, then start the procedure. Are you doing all right?" I nod. He looks toward the anesthesiologist, a tall, thin woman with creamy cocoa skin and the most perfect cheekbones I've ever seen. "Start her oxygen."

The anesthesiologist explains how the oxygen mask works as she slips it over my face. I feel smothered. I toss my head, gasp. "Relax," she says. "Relax. Breathe easy. Just breathe."

I calm my breathing. *It's oxygen, for goodness' sake. Calm down.* The oxygen irritates my nose. Burns.

"I shot a round on Sunday," a male voice says faintly. An instrument chinks as it's set down on a steel tray my blue tent shrouds from view.

"Where did you go?" someone asks.

"I played . . . perfect day to . . ." A machine beeps, measures my heart rate.

"Is that your regular course?" says another voice.

Calm. Stay calm. The woman with the perfect cheekbones looks down toward me, inspects, adjust knobs on equipment. The doctors begin to talk in murmurs. I can't hear their words. I also can't mistake their surprise. A sentence comes through clearly.

"Are you sure?"

That was Dr. McConaughey's voice. *Sure? Sure about what?* Silence. "Check again." More murmurs.

Dr. Randolph appears above the tent. "We took a quick cervical measurement, Darci. Quite a few, actually," he continues. "Your cervix is down to twenty millimeters." He shakes his head. "I . . . I . . . didn't think you'd lose this much cervix in two days."

He stuttered. My God. The unshakable Dr. Randolph just stuttered.

He rights himself, stands up tall, closes his lips. "Darci, we cannot do the Shirodkar cerclage. We have to do the MacDonald."

I think back to our first meeting, when he sewed his imaginary Shirodkar in the air, seeming superior to those other surgeons, the ones who do those lesser techniques.

"The MacDonald will be perfectly fine," he says. "There is not enough cervix left to do the Shirodkar." He pauses, looking toward me for some response. I say nothing as I lie here, helpless, speechless. "We'll get started," he says before disappearing from view.

The mask smothers me. I raise my hand and lift the mask from my face. The anesthesiologist leans down. "Can't breathe," I say, gulping air.

"You need to keep it on. Breathe slowly." She slips the mask back on. Holds my hand. Pats it gently.

"Let's push them up," Dr. Randolph says. Each of my leaden legs is grasped under the thigh, pushed toward my chest.

Splayed. My legs are held tight. Pressed harder. I can't breathe. There's intense pressure between my legs. The sensation isn't exactly pain, but foreign, wrong, like my flesh is being scooped out with a spoon. I can feel my flesh being whittled, mangled. I want to resist. Kick. Run. But my legs don't move, held captive with drugs, and hands.

The doctors resume talking golf. Two male voices discuss dogleg lefts and sand traps.

My chest tightens, my breath quick. Shallow. An alarm sounds from one of the monitors. I catch the anesthesiologist's eyes. She leans down and lifts the mask while I speak. "I'm scared," I confess, tears slipping down the sides of my face. I feel the violation of every push, every stitch.

She studies the monitor, then begins stroking my forehead. "You're okay," she says in long words that match the slow strokes of her hand. "It's all right." She pushes the surgical cap higher on my head, until the elastic reaches my hairline. Rubs my forehead with her thumb.

"Almost finished," Dr. Randolph says, out of sight. "Hang in there just a little longer."

I look up at the beautiful woman with the perfect cheekbones. Focus on the pinch of freckles scattered atop her cheeks. Focus on the gentle fingers. Ignore the pressure, the helplessness.

OCTOBER 25 *Thirteen weeks*

No answer. I've called his phone every ten minutes for over an hour. No answer. No returned call. Where are they?

Jon and Maddie left to do errands, have a little lunch. They were supposed to be back after lunch. It's nearly three. He's not here. I need to go to the hospital.

I didn't feel well. Queasy and feverish. Then I saw the discharge: yellow, foul. Something may be wrong. I called the doctor. The Saturday on-call doc said to go to the ER; it could be infection from the cerclage. I can't wait anymore. I give up on Jon, try Mary. Straight into voice mail. I call a neighbor for a ride. She doesn't know I'm pregnant. How do I nonchalantly ask for a ride to the emergency room?

"I'm sorry to bother you. But I can't reach Jon, and, well, I had a medical procedure this week. Minor. Only there's a small problem, and I need to go to the hospital."

Silence. "Do you want to go now?"

"Yes. I need to go in. Nothing major, I'm sure. Do you have time to take me?"

"I'm leaving now."

I scrawl a note for Jon. *At hospital. Check your voice mail.* I take deep breaths and try to ignore my sense of panic, try to focus on the hospital that's just moments away.

My neighbor rings the doorbell before I find my jacket.

~ ~ ~

"The stitches are intact," the ER doc says.

I lie on the exam table, dressed in a cotton hospital gown, knees bent, ankles pressed in stirrups, heart racing. The doctor widens the speculum, pinching my vaginal tract as the device expands.

"I see the discharge. It's around the stitches," she says. Then she inserts a swab, dabs for a sample, and releases the speculum.

"Do you think there's infection?"

"The surgical site does not look infected, but I can't say until the lab results are back."

"What about the discharge?"

"It could be your body's response to the stitches. Sometimes the body mounts an immune response, like the discharge you see. We should know in a few days. Until then, I'd like you to take an antibiotic." She grabs a pen from her jacket and begins scribbling on a scrip pad.

"Thank you. I'm glad to hear it's likely nothing, but I had to be sure. I was just so frightened, when I saw the discharge . . ." I drop my head, trying not to think about my twins, the strange discharge that started the day before I lost them. I still wonder what might have happened if I'd gone to the hospital then, called the doctor about the discharge. And I am ground to a nub from the ever-present anxiety of this pregnancy, eviscerated by the perils that seem constant, uncontrollable, and familiar.

"Go home. Get back in bed." The doctor says she'll send someone with discharge papers.

I sit for a minute before dressing. My lip quivers as I pull the red sweatshirt over my head. I walk toward the hospital exit, shoulders slumped, arms crossed. The automatic doors swoosh open as I make my way outside. The neighbor is gone. A dozen cars clog the circular driveway. Toward the end, I see a cab, rare in this suburban community. I walk toward it before hearing Jon's voice, then his footsteps racing up the sidewalk.

He clutches me in his arms. "What happened? Is everything okay?"

We walk toward the car while I tell him what the doctor said. "And where were you?" I hiss, fear suddenly taking a backseat to anger.

"I'm sorry. I forgot my cell phone. I never got your calls. Then I saw the note." I am silent and Jon's contrite the whole way home.

~ ~ ~

The room swirls out of focus. The man in the center remains clear, crisp, wrapped in pale green scrubs, black eyes barely visible between his surgical mask and cap.

"Give me the baby."

I turn my head, ignore his insistence. I'm hot. Can't somebody open a window?

"Stay with me. Darci. Darci!" he screams, not allowing the escape of unconsciousness again. "I need your permission." His eyes squint, the folds of his puckered brow slipping beneath the surgical cap. "I have to take the baby."

"I won't let you have her." How dare he. Her heart is beating. Doesn't he see the monitor? So hot.

"Fever is a sign of infection. This is serious. Darci, you have to let me take the BABY."

"NO."

I awake trembling, covered in sweat. For a moment I was back there. In the hospital room. Again. If only I could tell myself it was never real—but it was.

I slip from bed while Jon sleeps, into the hall bathroom. I light a candle, turn on the water, hot. Steam fills the room while I step into the shower and then lean toward the white tiled wall, resting my lowered head against my forearm. The heat beats against my back. I tilt my head back, soaking my hair. Hot water drips down my face and mixes with tears. I start to sob loudly. I want to be quiet, to let everyone sleep. But my fear becomes illustrated in dreams, vivid recollections of the experience all too real, all too unforgettable. I awake numb and frightened, left to another day spent wondering if I'll ever hold this baby.

I turn off the water, lift my head to step out. Jon sits, head down, holding a towel for me.

➤ OCTOBER 28

I hear Jon and Maddie's laughter from the side yard where they play. I'm inside, trying to bury my thoughts in the newspaper, barely able to follow the straightforward style of *USA Today*. My mind keeps drifting back to my first miscarriage, lost at thirteen weeks gestation more than four years ago.

I panicked at the sight of blood when I rose for work that morning. Instead of going to my office, we raced to the obstetrician. An ultrasound quickly confirmed that I was losing my pregnancy, and that our baby had stopped developing weeks earlier. I was only starting to bleed now because my body finally recognized that the baby was lost.

The doctor said not to worry, that these things just happen. She then sent me home to miscarry naturally, without a D&C. I cried and cramped and seethed in an anguish that grew as every dribble slipped from my body, waiting for the blood to stop, wondering what I would see before this was all over. After a week I carried my physical pain and emotional torment back to my obstetrician's office, begging her to make this stop. She then performed a D&C.

I asked how this could have happened, especially at thirteen weeks, when the chance of miscarriage had largely passed. Could something possibly be wrong? I'd already had one baby twelve weeks premature, and now I was losing my second pregnancy. After a week of sitting with the reality that the child I'd imagined would never be, I felt numb and damaged, and reeled from a future once thought ensured, now turned uncertain. I asked about testing to look for causes of my loss.

"This is only your first miscarriage," she said. "It's probably nature's way of taking care of an abnormal pregnancy. It's unlikely that anything is wrong."

Her response didn't feel right. Doctors are scientists; how can they willingly accept mere likelihood when confirmation is available? I pressed the issue and insisted on chromosome analysis of my lost baby. The test came back weeks later; the results were inconclusive, meaning that we could not determine whether the baby's chromosomes were normal or abnormal.

I cried for my baby, usually at night, sitting alone in a chair while Jon and Maddie slept. Even after months had passed, I could not stop thinking about my loss. Was it my fault? Would we ever build the family we'd imagined? Was something wrong with me that caused my miscarriage?

The doctor discouraged further testing, reminding me that it was only one loss. I deferred to her authority, and returned to endless days and sleepless nights in which culpability and uncertainty lingered. At the time, I didn't know about medical standards that exclude testing until multiple miscarriages. I also didn't know that the longer a pregnancy develops, the lower the odds of chromosome errors. When a loss happens after ten weeks gestation, the odds of chromosome abnormalities are thought to be only 5 percent.[15]

Had I known, I would have insisted on further testing after my first loss at thirteen weeks. And if I had, I would likely be running through the yard with my children instead of waiting on this couch, hoping I don't lose this child, longing for the babies that only still exist in my mind.

~ OCTOBER 31 *Fourteen weeks*

"Say Happy Halloweeeeen." Jon snaps the camera and my eyes see glowing shadows.

"You look gorgeous, girl." I take in Maddie, dressed as a mermaid with green satin gills and cotton seashells covering her chest.

"You look good, too. You're the best Snow White ever."

I couldn't stand the idea of staying inside on Halloween. Jon and I often dress up, one year as matching cows, another as a Girl Scout and a Boy Scout, with Jon wearing a leather backpack to further his authenticity. And I can't imagine missing the tiny devils and princesses with their expectant grins as they grab their treats. I felt crushed at the thought of missing them, and then I thought of Snow White, lying fast asleep after the poisoned apple, awaiting her prince.

In this costume my bed rest doesn't have to feel awkward or isolating. One of the most difficult parts of all this is missing the world around me, and when I do interact with people, I occasionally hear some dolt offering their critical evaluation of the tough choices I've had to make.

After I lost my twins despite twelve weeks of bed rest, one woman repeatedly told me the same story of how her doctor recommended bed rest, but how she ignored the advice and had a successful pregnancy anyway—as if I'd been a fool to ever follow such guidance. Others denounced our choice to keep trying after so many losses, never understanding that when I walk into my dining room, I always see the empty seats at my table.

Halloween offers a chance to participate in the world without the risk of unsolicited judgment. I'm grateful to be breathing fresh air as just another costumed character instead of an immobilized woman, tethered to a bed.

For my big night out, the front porch is transformed into Snow's comatose scene. I recline on a toddler bed draped with a green silk duvet cover, my feet spilling onto a patio chair. A basket of apples lies on its side, contents strewn across the porch. My itchy rayon costume, a long gold and blue gown with a red cape, looks just like the book cover that rests at my feet. The hair is another story. A large red bow sits atop a cheap black wig that looks mangled, like it was chewed by a dog. I do look like Snow White, but maybe after she's had a few too many.

I wave as Maddie's red curls sway when she waddles away in the snug mermaid bottom, wondering whether I'll be joining her next year with a tiny bundle dressed as a little pumpkin or sleeping goblin.

NOVEMBER

⬣ NOVEMBER 1 *Fourteen weeks*

"You look great today." Mary sits in the armchair adjacent to the couch, now my daybed heaped with blankets.

I lean up on the sofa and run fingers through my hair, tucking the sides behind my ears. I haven't seen anything close to makeup in weeks, and my hair hasn't been washed in two days. Mary is a true friend. Not only did she smuggle real, caffeinated coffee into my cell this morning, but she's willing to tell a tiny motivational lie when needed. "Well, these are my good sweats. Thank you."

"What's going on this week? Did you see any of your doctors?"

I sip my coffee, the first caffeine I've had since August, and revel in the rebellion. "I saw Dr. Randolph a few days ago." I tell her the good news first: I was able to restart heparin last week, reducing the threat from Factor V Leiden and easing my mind. "But with my delinquent cervix at twenty millimeters, I need to stay on bed rest." It feels strange, knowing that this part of me is defective in such objective terms, but I feel fortunate that I know. At least I have the chance to try to do something about it.

Whether a woman's cervix is ever measured during pregnancy depends on her doctor. Even among high-risk patients, some doctors question the value of these measurements and do not take them. Others swear by their utility. During the only ultrasound for my pregnancy with Maddie, the test facility took a cervical measurement. I didn't ask; it was simply that hospital's standard procedure: Every patient gets a cervical measurement whenever a Level II ultrasound is completed. When I had the Level II ultrasound for my twins at a different hospital, just two weeks before their loss, no cervical measurement was taken. It was not standard procedure for that facility to look at the cervix. It's no additional work to take the measurement when already doing a vaginal ultrasound, yet some facilities choose to, and others choose not to. The choice is rarely made by the pregnant women who don't understand the potential value of this information and don't know that they need to ask.

"I wonder how my mom dealt with all this when she was pregnant with me. I mean, she knew she had a problem; the doctor reinforced her cervix." She takes one last bite of cinnamon roll, popping a finger in her mouth for the last bits of icing. "But that was it. She didn't have measurements, nothing to let her know how things were going."

"I think I'd go crazy without the number. It's not great right now, but at least I know." I tell her about the studies that tie short cervical length to preterm delivery, and then grab a second scone from the plate.

"How about Jon? Does he follow all the numbers too, gobble up all the research he can get?"

How I wish that were the case. He doesn't look at the studies. His body stiffens and he finds an excuse to leave the room whenever I bring it up. Jon is highly involved in this pregnancy—caring for me, coming to most appointments—but when it comes to staring down the research, I do that alone.

Parts of this pregnancy have felt desolate, as did parts of my losses. Women often suffer gaping emotional wounds after a miscarriage; spouses try to understand, but for many, the experience is too intangible to make a deep impact. These disparate experiences can tear marriages apart, leaving women feeling distant from their husbands. And how could women not feel this way? The logical consequence of pain borne in isolation can only be distance.

I know these gaps. We've worked to close them after the tragedies that dissolved me and eventually left Jon impatient with my grief after months of recovery drained his initial support.

"He likes the measurements. But he doesn't like to look at the other stuff—the books, the research." I think back to the therapy sessions after Maddie's premature birth, then after the first miscarriage at thirteen weeks. The therapist said that men and women deal with loss differently. It's not realistic for couples to expect an identical experience, but it's necessary for each person to work through loss in their own way, with support and understanding from their spouse. "He deals with all this in his own way."

I've come to accept that while Jon suffered from our losses, his pain generated a different response than mine. Despite this acceptance, his unwillingness to engage in the research somehow reopens the old wounds when I interpreted his divergent reaction as an indictment against what I felt, a silent admonishment against what I needed to heal.

Mary picks up a book, *Preventing Miscarriage: The Good News*, from atop the pile that rests on the coffee table. This is the first book I ever read about causes of pregnancy loss, and the pages are filled with highlights and notes flagging portions I believed relevant to me. These pages planted the seeds that cultivated my own research efforts that eventually led to my diagnosis.

She flips through the pages. "I see this out a lot. Is this one of your favorites?"

NOVEMBER 5

"The cerclage looks good. There's some pus around the stitches, but it still looks intact." The speculum pinches a moment longer before Dr. McConaughey releases the device. *It's intact.* I hold on to these words, trying to blight the phrase my mind adds to his sentence: *for now.*

"How do we know it will continue to hold?" I imagine my body as a broken vase, frailly adhered with glue, dreading the next jarring blow. Jon stops reading and sits up in his chair.

"What was your last cervical measurement with Dr. Randolph?" Dr. McConaughey opens my file to scan for the data point.

"Twenty millimeters, seven days ago," I answer, before he finds the page. At 20 millimeters, *normal* women have a 20 percent likelihood of preterm birth or pregnancy loss. For women who already have histories of premature birth and loss—we "high-risk" women—the risk is likely even greater.

"What are the odds this won't work?" Jon sets his *Newsweek* on the floor.

"Each case is unique, but cerclage prevents preterm delivery in a majority of cases." Dr. McConaughey speaks while turning pages in my file. "It was twenty millimeters when we did your cerclage in October. Cervical length is stable. That's a good sign."

I nod. Not because he has allayed my fears, but because I feel bad for him. How often does he face women like me, still tormented by unforgettable experiences, asking unanswerable questions?

"One last issue." Dr. McConaughey closes the file. "Have you discussed an amniocentesis with Dr. Randolph?"

"We don't want to do an amnio with this pregnancy," Jon says. "We don't want to add more risk."

"Dr. Randolph set us up for integrated screening. If the numbers look good we won't do anything invasive."

"He said the tests can come back great—like only one chance in thousands that there's a problem." Jon looks as though the encouraging results were already in his hands.

Dr. McConaughey stares at Jon. "Sometimes." He gives a quick nod before leaving.

Jon smiles as he hands me my sweats. He has seemed less stressed since we found regular child care, reducing his burden to merely crazed instead of unmanageable. When he gives me my shirt, he pokes my belly, and I think he expects me to giggle.

I glower.

"What's wrong?" he says.

"What's wrong? Are you joking?"

He steps back.

"We can't be sure the cerclage is going to hold. My cervix is already shortened and I'm only fourteen weeks. Now I get to go home and stab myself with medicine that may not even help. And you ask me what's wrong?"

"I thought we just had a great office visit."

I pull on my shirt, remind myself that he is here, with me, trying to help. "So tell me what you think was so great about it."

He pauses. "Well, the cerclage is still holding. That's good."

"Okay."

"And you haven't lost any more cervix. The number is stable." As we talk about these indicators, I'm amazed by his ability to let these few immediate points assuage the entirety of our reality—a reality he escapes through work and distraction, but one I live with continually.

This reminds me of Maddie's stay in the NICU. Jon told himself that Maddie was a healthy baby who just needed to live in the hospital for a while. He went to work every day, then visited her every night, laughing with the nurses, finding something to smile at while she lay connected to tubes and machines in her incubator. I sat by her most of the day, witnessing the times she stopped breathing, the alarms that blared ominous warnings. He stayed busy. I eventually stayed medicated.

"Jon, it's like we're having two separate experiences, hearing completely different things." And how could we not be? He's never read any of the research. He hears *Twenty millimeters: stable cervical length;* I hear *Twenty millimeters: high chance of preterm labor.* "Let's go home. I want you to look at one of the studies about cervical length."

He shakes his head.

"You need to see this study. The methodology was rock solid and the correlation with shorter lengths and loss—"

"NO." He stares with pupils so wide they devour the green of his eyes. We stand, silently, as his chest rises and falls with growing force.

I reach over, grab his hand. My jaw softens as I grasp his

fingers and honor the space he needs, reminding myself that despite our different ways of dealing with all of this, he is here, with me.

NOVEMBER 13 *Sixteen weeks*

"Just a little stick." I turn my head as Dr. Randolph inserts the needle, still reluctant to watch my skin being pierced, despite months of self-injection. After the needle is secure, I watch as the blood fills the tube. I'm unfazed by the sight of blood, but still agitated after the prick of the needle. "This is the last of the integrated screening tests," he says.

"When should we know something?" Jon hovers over me, studying the blood that fills the vial as though he might see any abnormalities lurking in the tube.

"We'll know early next week." Dr. Randolph caps off the first vial and puts on a second empty tube. Then a third.

"Dr. Randolph, were you happy with the number today?" Jon asks.

"Rather reassuring. I was glad to see the cervix at thirty-three millimeters." The doctor reminds us that my cervix may change during the coming months. In normal pregnancies, significant shortening doesn't happen before later in the third trimester. In some cases when the cervix shortens too early, it can correct itself.

"I've read that it's around this time—fifteen or sixteen weeks—that most losses from cervical incompetence happen." I lean forward in the chair. "Is that true?"

"It is common to see losses at this point. But they can also happen later."

"Does our measurement mean we're out of the woods, at least for now?" Jon leans closer.

"No. The cervix appears stable at the moment. That's a good sign. But as you've already seen, the cervix is dynamic, and these measurements are only a possible indicator of preterm labor. We need to remain quite cautious."

"But it is encouraging, at least for now." Jon waits. The doctor shoots him a nonresponsive look before my husband looks toward me and smiles. After the fourth tube of blood is drawn, we head for the elevator.

"I think that was an eight." Jon pushes the down button.

"What was an eight?"

"The office visit. On a scale of one to ten, with ten being great, I left there feeling like an eight." He looks serious, but pleased. The elevator opens to the lobby. "I've been thinking about what you said, how we seem to hear things differently. Maybe it would help if we rate ourselves after appointments. You know, figure out that we're in different places before we blow up."

"Eight?" I take in my husband, appreciating his effort to ease our tension. "That sounds about right for today."

He squeezes my hand before leaving me on the bench to get the car.

 ⟳ NOVEMBER 18

"I have your integrated screening results."

I sit up in bed and grab the legal pad atop the nightstand, clenching the phone between my ear and shoulder. "Go ahead, Dr. Randolph."

"It's not bad, but not exactly what we'd hoped. The chance

of Down syndrome is 1 in 170." He pauses. "The likelihood of any chromosome abnormality is about 1 in 90."

I write down the numbers, shaking my head. "Not the 1 in 3,000 or 4,000 we'd hoped for."

"Keep in mind, these tests are only indicators, not diagnostic tests." He again stresses that whether the odds came back one in two, or one in a million, these tests do not conclusively determine chromosome status. "Only CVS or amniocentesis can do that."

"What do you recommend?"

"Of course, you need not do any further testing. But with the results offering only marginal improvement over your age-related odds, you should consider an amnio."

I drop my head, put down the pen. "Jon and I need to talk it over. I'll call you tomorrow."

~ ~ ~

"I think we need to do it." Jon leans against the fireplace, sliding his hand over his lips.

I sit up on the sofa, straightening out the down comforter covering my legs. "I hate this. I didn't want to have to do this again."

We never intended to have an amnio with Maddie. I was only thirty-one, carrying my first pregnancy, still untouched by all the losses to come. The pregnancy felt surreal, as if we didn't really get that we'd have a baby, a tiny person to be protected, nurtured. We put off the recommended ultrasound until nineteen weeks—and then went only for "baby pictures," not to quiet the possibility that something could be wrong. When the ultrasound technician became silent and excused herself to get a doctor, that's when reality came into focus.

The baby has cysts in her brain.

What . . . how . . .

. . . correlates with a chromosome abnormality that causes vital organs to fail.

What happens to these babies?

Most never leave the hospital. The others die before their first birthday.

The doctor whisked us into the procedure room for an amnio. I watched through an ultrasound while the long needle pierced my stomach, penetrated my baby's sac, and sucked up the telltale fluid that would reveal her future. We waited eleven days before getting the results; eleven days fearing that Maddie was fated for death before her first birthday.

And then there were my twins, lost two weeks after an amniocentesis. Despite the discovery of the clotting disorder and the diagnosis of cervical incompetence, a shard of question lingers.

"Do you not want to do it?" Jon asks, sitting down beside me.

I shrug. "I think we have to. I don't think I can take any more unknowns." I'm not sure what we'd do if the results revealed a serious problem, but I feel a compelling need to know, a need to have insight into a future that feels threatened from all sides.

"Shit. What happened to those minuscule odds? The chance of getting numbers that looked like one in thousands instead of one in a few hundred? Why couldn't we get those numbers?"

〜 NOVEMBER 19

"You have to push." The resident's now-pale face is contorted with frustration, hair disheveled. When I got to the hospital at midnight last night, leaking amniotic fluid, twenty weeks pregnant with twins, this resident refused to call an experienced doctor. At this hospital, the residents run

the whole show in maternity, she had said, beaming with pride, as though her résumé should be my primary concern.

"I did push. Nothing's happening." *The resident looks at the monitor that graphs the crests and troughs of my contractions. The line is rising. My stomach feels firmer, like I'm doing crunches, but not painful.*

"Come on. You have to push. The baby has to come out."

"It's not working. He's just not coming." *What does she mean, push him out? He's only twenty weeks. He'll stay here. With me.*

Jon stands close to my hospital bed, wired, terrified, speechless. The resident paces the room, stops to speak in hushed tones to a nurse. Then Dr. D walks in.

"I'm so glad you're here." *Jon dissolves toward our regular obstetrician.*

"Darci, I'm sorry to see you back here." *The doctor shakes his head, no doubt thinking about seeing me just yesterday, when I thought something was wrong, when he sent me home.*

When I paged him at noon, he met me at the ER, coming back from a holiday, to personally care for his patient. He had heard my twins' strong and steady heartbeats; he had tested the strange discharge and said it was not amniotic fluid; he had performed a pelvic exam, which showed no external signs of dilation. He then reassured me that my babies were fine before mentioning one additional test: an ultrasound to confirm no internal signs of labor. He believed the ultrasound was unnecessary, but was willing to do it if I needed more proof to allay my fears. I had studied my trusted, seemingly infallible, obstetrician, and deferred to his judgment.

Would I be here now if I had insisted on the ultrasound? Would we have seen that labor was imminent before I began seeping amniotic fluid?

"Dr. D, what's going on?" *I rise to my elbows.*

"You are leaking amniotic fluid from the lower twin's sac."

"My son, Dr. D. You mean my son's sac."

"Yes. From the male."

"How can this be happening? I just saw you yesterday. You said my cervix was closed. You said everything was fine."

"I don't know what happened." He hangs his head.

"But when I came in last night with the back pain, the leaking, they gave me drugs, inverted my feet higher than my head . . ."

"They tried to stop your contractions. But your cervix is well dilated. You are in labor."

"I know my son is in distress. But what can we do?"

"There's nothing more we can do."

"But his heart is beating. I saw when we came in last night. I know it's gotten weaker . . ."

"Darci, his heart is no longer beating. He is gone."

"There's a heartbeat on the monitor." I point to the machine, hear its bleeps, see the lines jump.

"That is the female. The male has no heartbeat."

I turn away from the monitor. Jon grasps my hand.

"Darci, we need to take the babies. They need to come out."

"No. I can't. They're just twenty weeks. They can't come yet." He can't be gone. There must be something. And her. She's not gone. "Her heart is beating. You just said so. You can't take her."

"When we lose one twin, it's rare to save the other. And there is great risk for the mother."

"What's the risk?" Jon steps closer.

"There is a high risk of infection for—"

"I won't let you take her." I stare and Dr. D looks away.

~ ~ ~

"Push. Bear down," the doctor commands.

I grunt. Yell. Grip the rails of the hospital bed. "He's not coming. Can't."

"He has to come out. I need you to push."

I can't. I won't. How can I push him out into a world with no place for him?

"Darci, he is gone. He has to come out. This is our only chance to save the other baby. You have to push."

No. God, no.

"Once he's out, we can try to stop your labor. We can try to save her. But there is a high risk for infection. Are you sure you don't want me to take them both?"

"NO! Please. Please. I need to save her."

"Then you need to push. Now."

"How can I do this to my son?"

"He is gone. Darci, He Is Gone."

Oh, God. I have to push him out but how can I do this how can I let go of the baby I need to protect. Grip the rails. Scream. Oh, God! Push until I begin to shake. The phone starts to ring.

"Good. PUSH."

I scream through gritted teeth and the phone keeps ringing.

"All right. Keep pushing. Push."

Tremble. Ring. Ring. My head may explode from the pressure and my gripped hands are white. Ring. Ring.

"Stay with it. Come on."

Pushhh. Pushhh. Ring. That fucking phone. Let go of the rails. "STOP IT! JUST STOP!" *I scream toward the phone.*

The resident grabs the phone, rips the cord from the wall.

I fall back into the bed. Close my eyes. Drift away.

"Darci. No! Stay with me. You need to push." *Dr. D stands above me, yelling, forbidding the escape of unconsciousness.*

Jon stands by my bed, face white, hands pressed to his cheeks. A nurse walks out of the room. Dr. D steps toward the end of my bed. The heart rate monitors bleep. Mine. Hers.

I'm so sorry, little boy.

Grab the rails. Push. Grit my teeth.

Please forgive me, my precious prince.

Pushhh. Can't let up.

I love you. I swear I do.

Pushhh. Scream.

Something gives. Slowly. Faster. Sliding through my body and I have to see. I need to look at him and let him know his mother's gaze just once. I thrust forward.

The room goes black.

I scream out. Bolt up in the dampened bed in the darkened room.

"What? What! Is there pain?" Jon rips himself from sleep and slides his hand across the wet pajamas that cling to my back.

"The babies. Oh, God! Our babies."

The fear in his face turns to recognition. I then see our shared anguish in his eyes. "I know. I know." He strokes my hair as we rock back and forth. "I miss them, too," he whispers.

 NOVEMBER 24 *Seventeen weeks*

"Everything looks good. Exactly what we would expect to find," Dr. Randolph says.

Despite his tensed face, Jon strokes my arm while Dr. Randolph continues with the full fetal anatomy scan. I become mindful of my own puckered forehead and cinched nose and try to smooth them, wondering to what degree Jon's tension mirrors my own.

"Does the brain look normal? With Maddie, there were cysts . . ." Jon trails off.

Dr. Randolph repositions the ultrasound transducer and

studies the monitor. "There are no visible cysts." He examines the baby's head a few more minutes as if to reaffirm his statement. Then his expression turns pleasant, almost playful. "Do you want to know the sex of the baby?"

"NO." We speak in unison, unrehearsed but aligned against a degree of tangibility we need to hold distant.

Dr. Randolph quickly dissolves back into his expressionless mold.

We know the baby's vital organs look fine: a four-chambered heart, two kidneys, a healthy liver. The umbilical cord has three vessels with normal blood flow. The baby's head and nuchal fold measure within expected ranges. All indicators suggest that this baby is okay. But we need something closer to certainty, not mere suggestion.

"Alrighty," Dr. Randolph says. "Let's get started with the amnio."

His assistant places a thin plastic package on a stainless steel tray covered with dimpled cloth while Dr. Randolph splatters warm gel on my stomach. He presses the abdominal transducer against my skin, moving it with wide motions, then smaller, tiny corrections before settling on a spot. "Hold it here, at this angle." His assistant takes the transducer, holds it in place.

"I'm using a twenty-two-gauge needle," he says, opening the package. This could be the longest needle I've ever seen. The size is necessary to puncture my skin, pass through layers of abdominal fat, penetrate the uterine wall, and, finally, pierce the protective sac that holds my baby. "The needle is not very thick, so it leaves just a nick in the sac."

He nods. I shoot back a blank stare.

Dr. Randolph signals to his assistant and points to a spot on my belly. My stomach feels damp and cool as she wipes the area with a wet cotton pad. Jon squeezes my hand and bites his lip as he watches.

"The ultrasound lets us see the needle going in. We can be certain to keep it away from the baby, make sure we only get what we intend," Dr. Randolph reassures. "Ready?"

"Yes." I take a deep breath.

The needle breaks through my skin. I grasp the edge of the exam table and lie perfectly still, ignoring the pressure and stinging sear that doesn't subside. The needle slides through my fat with deliberate, thoughtful motion. No quick jab. The placement must be precise. I watch the ultrasound screen as a thin black spear emerges into view, grows longer and longer until it rests.

Dr. Randolph holds the needle delicately, easing up the plunger. "We want to take . . . as little fluid . . . as possible." The vacuum begins to fill with clear liquid. I look toward the monitor, hoping the baby doesn't move. What if my baby jumps, punctures an arm or a leg on the tiny dagger, jabs an eye or an ear?

After a few minutes, Dr. Randolph removes the needle. Surgical tape screeches from a roll before the nurse dresses the wound. Dr. Randolph holds the vial up toward the light.

"We drew about eighteen milliliters of fluid." He pauses and turns the vial to examine it from another angle. "The fluid looks clear. And there was no contact with the baby." He audibly exhales.

"When do we get the results?" Jon asks.

Dr. Randolph explains that the test usually takes ten to fourteen days. "In the meantime, I want you to call me with any bleeding or cramping, okay?" His face reveals a level of concern always apparent in his attentiveness, but rarely visible.

I nod. "Thank you, Dr. Randolph."

NOVEMBER 25

I lie in bed, flat, where I've been since coming home from the ultrasound yesterday. I haven't risked any excursions down to the couch. The first few days after the amnio are the most crucial, when the sac works to allay the wound left by the needle. There is no cramping, no bleeding, no unexplained discharge— all signs that would likely come if something were wrong. I have no idea whether my added caution is necessary, but I know it can't hurt; and if something goes wrong, I'll be spared the anguish of second-guessing my every movement after the procedure. I don't know how I would deal with the bigger issue, the culpability that comes with electing to have done the procedure.

"Surprise!" Jon and Maddie shout. Jon carries bags of takeout stacked atop Maddie's toddler play table held against his chest. Maddie follows, beaming, carrying two wooden toddler chairs. The room quickly fills with the unmistakable smell of Broasted chicken.

"What's all this?"

Jon places the eighteen-inch-tall table on the floor, adjacent to my bed. "We thought we would all eat up here tonight, since you can't come down." He begins pulling food containers from paper bags and stacking them on the square wooden tabletop. There's Broasted chicken from a newly discovered takeout shack, mashed potatoes and roasted vegetables from Whole Foods, and a box of cookies from the bakery down the street.

"This looks amazing. And you went to so much trouble. This was quite a few stops."

"We wanted to get you all your favorites." Maddie puffs out her chest and grins wildly. She and Jon pull the toddler chairs up to the toddler table and start loading up plates.

Maddie still looks right seated at the table we bought for her at two. Jon . . . not so much. His six-foot-tall, hundred-and-eighty-pound frame has swallowed the pint-sized chair, and he struggles to get his runner's legs under, or around, or beside the miniature table.

I take a bite of chicken, warm, and juice drips to my chin as the skin crunches under my teeth. The flavor is rich, salty, heaven. I smile at my husband with grease-glistened lips.

"I wanted to do something nice for you. I know you're having a hard time." His eyes are wide as I look down at him from our oversized sleigh bed. I lean down and he rises to kiss me.

＞ NOVEMBER 27 *Eighteen weeks*

"What else do you need?" My mother-in-law places another fresh pitcher of ice water on the nightstand, removing the old one with cubes still melting, pushing aside the magazines she piled on just this morning.

I've barely seen Jon since Steve and Ev came yesterday for the holiday weekend. "Nothing. I'm so fine right now."

"You want some food? Steve won't have your dinner for another hour," she says, referring to the homemade Asian feast of vegetable spring rolls with three dipping sauces, marinated five-spice chicken, and sautéed bok choy, red peppers, and broccoli in a red chili sauce. "He's making all your favorites, you know."

"I know. He makes me feel so special."

"That's because you are special." She smiles and leans in to tousle my hair. "I could bring you some pot roast from last night."

"No thanks." On the surface, you'd never know my mother-in-law was a doting parent and grandma. Her thin athletic build and wispy dark updo scream more trophy wife than devoted partner of more than forty years. And once, before Jon and I went away for a weekend, she tried to talk me into getting a temporary tattoo.

It'll be fun. Something different.

I don't think so.

Come on. Why not try it?

I don't know.

At least think about it.

Okay. I'll think about it.

Good. Good.

"I know what I wanted to ask you," she says, pulling up the dining room chair that Steve carried up when they arrived. "Did you read the front page of today's *Times*?" We discuss the article on adding a prescription benefit to Medicare from today's *New York Times*. It dawns on me that she's nearly old enough to qualify for Medicare.

We talk about the Florida senate race. Then the latest from *People* about Bennifer. I'm so grateful for the company. Because I went on bed rest just weeks after moving here, I never had a chance to make new friends. Mary is my only regular visitor.

"Tell me, Darci. How are you doing? For real."

"I'm good . . . I mean, you guys are taking such good care of me, I—"

"Emotionally. How are you doing emotionally?"

I lean up in bed and prop pillows farther down my shoulders. "Well. I'm . . . scared." Do I tell her about the dread that each phone call may be a bad amnio result? The nightmares that recur with increasing frequency? The continuing torment of yearning for the four children I've already lost, and wondering whether this baby will be added to the list of thwarted lives?

I look toward this woman, who was with me within hours of Maddie's birth, with me during the first miscarriage, with me after I lost my precious twins. Her eyes moisten and her fists clench.

"But I know we're doing everything we can. And I'm holding on to that."

She shakes her head, bites her lip.

"We're getting every possible treatment, giving this baby every possible chance. There's no reason to think that this time can't be different. Better." I nod, trying to believe my own words.

"Absolutely. This time will be fine. Just fine." She strokes my arm before leaving the room, returning in minutes with a heaping plate of pot roast.

DECEMBER

I stare at the clock: 1:08 P.M. In minutes I will pick up the phone and dial my old therapist in California for our phone session. I first saw Dr. Geffen when Maddie was in the NICU. After weeks of watching my three-pound daughter struggle, first on a respirator, then her entire head wrapped in a gauzy mask that forced oxygen into her lungs, then trying, and sometimes failing, to breathe on her own, my eyes twitched and my hands shook. A nurse asked me to see Dr. Geffen, a psychologist who regularly worked with the mothers of preemies.

She has helped me through each loss over the past six years. Still, when I speak with her, it's always a mixed blessing of discomfort and insight. My stomach knots with nervous queasiness, like I'm about to enter a church confessional.

At exactly ten past one I dial the phone. She's always been a stickler about being just on time, and I doubt her rules have relaxed in the year since I last saw her, when I crumbled after losing my twins. The phone rings just twice. "Mrs. Klein, I was surprised when I got your message."

Mrs. Klein. I hate when she calls me Mrs. Klein. I've asked her to use my first name. She won't—says it usurps my authority if she addresses me on such informal terms. But isn't it usurping my authority when she refuses to do what I've asked?

"Dr. Geffen, thank you for agreeing to do a phone session. I'm going a little crazy here, given the circumstances." *Did I just say "crazy" to a therapist?* I shake my head before telling her about the bleeding, the low heart rate, the cerclage, and my dwindling cervix. I confess my fears for Maddie, the intermittent conflicts with Jon. Then I get around to the real reason I called: the pervasive fear that something will go hopelessly wrong with this pregnancy.

"I wake up every day with the same question: Is this the day I'll lose my baby?" There. I've said it. There's some relief in the admission, but what can she really do? How can realistic fears be diminished?

"Of course you're anxious. With your history, and what you've just described, who wouldn't be?"

I know I'm entitled to my fears, but somehow hearing the words from her further validates my anxiety. It seems like a simple idea—women who've lost babies are scared and anxious during their next pregnancy—but unless people have lived through it, they don't seem to get it. When I chat with friends who've known this pain, they always ask how I'm holding up, and we talk about the fear; the others never bring it up.

Multiple studies have confirmed that pregnant women who've had a loss experience far more anxiety during future pregnancies than those who've never miscarried.[16,17,18] After loss, women must push aside the constant whisper that things could go wrong again. In my case, the message comes in more of a scream.

"I'm having nightmares. Dr. Geffen, I've started to relive it." I hold the headset in place and scoot farther down in bed, pulling blankets high over my shoulders. "I relive every moment of losing my twins when I sleep."

"How often do you have these dreams?"

"Every few days. They started maybe three weeks ago."

"And how far along are you in this pregnancy?"

I pause, realizing the significance of her question. "Eighteen weeks."

"So you're approaching twenty weeks, the point when you lost your twins."

Silence. I sit up in bed, shift my eyes among the corners of the room.

"The anniversary of loss can be agonizing, Mrs. Klein." She says that my mind is bound to mark each week in the pregnancy, draw parallels between past losses and now, especially around the time of loss. "It's natural that your fears would spike at this time, even if you weren't having such a difficult pregnancy. And the fact that you're confined to bed is bound to make it even worse."

I drop my head into my hands. "I know it would help if I could go out, do some yoga, get some exercise. But I'm stuck here in bed. What can I do?"

"Try to calm yourself as much as you can. I know it's hard, but you need to reduce some of the stress of your pregnancy."

We talk about breathing techniques and meditation. She asked me to read several books on mindfulness years ago, writings about being present in the current moment, releasing all the pain of the past to cultivate the possibility of what's real, now, in this moment.

"But Dr. Geffen, I don't really want to be present in this moment. That's why I'm calling you. This is all too damn scary."

"That's the fear talking, from all the past losses, all the old pain. And it is a legitimate part of who you are. I am not telling you to ignore it, but isn't there something else that exists today?"

I stop to think, look at the ceiling, and then glance at the floor.

"Isn't there some hope? At this moment, your body is creating life, protecting the baby that you have spent years fighting for."

I take a deep breath. "Yes, yes it is."

"So that's also a part of your reality, right?"

I close my eyes and hold my stomach, caress my skin with my thumb. "Yes."

"Mrs. Klein, don't misunderstand what I am saying. I'm not implying that this should be easy. Your situation is extremely difficult. But if you can be mindful—let the fear come, but don't judge it—then it will move through you. You can't wish it away, or ignore it; you need to sit with your fear until it's ready to leave."

I remember this advice. I heard it after I lost my twins, when the anguish of past losses accumulated to an omnipresent fear that ruthlessly crushed my very essence. At first I was eager to cry and scream and pour it all out, as though I could rush through all the grief and be done with the sorrow. I wanted to push it all away and get back to my old life. That would have been a mistake.

Dr. Geffen convinced me that I needed to sit with my grief, let it come and go as it pleased, that this was the only way to truly move past my tragedies and return to my life without the overwhelming shadow of loss ever present.

I wept for months. I journaled and examined everything I felt. And then I found myself crying less frequently; not because I held it back, but because the grief had begun to move away. I was making peace with my losses.

"Allow yourself to feel the fear instead of fighting the emotion. As it starts to move through you, there'll be more mental space for other things." Dr. Geffen pauses while I consider her advice. "You may even find yourself connecting to the joy of your pregnancy, and all the possibility it brings."

"I do feel some joy, Dr. Geffen. There are moments when I can let go of the risk, the whole situation, and just have fun with Jon and Maddie. But it's getting harder to connect with any joy right now. The fear is pervasive—sometimes so relentless I don't think I can take it anymore."

"When you can't stay with it any longer, try distracting yourself. Distraction is a short-term solution, but when you need some temporary relief, there's nothing wrong with it."

I look around the floor and survey my paltry tools of distraction: stacks of books and magazines, my computer, a journal to scribe my thoughts and fears. Then I look out the window, where a clear winter sky makes even the barren branches look a brilliant shade of gray. I take a deep breath and glimpse myself next winter, strolling my bundled baby under a dazzling winter blue sky that makes both our faces glisten.

～ DECEMBER 6 *Nineteen weeks*

"That's the third time I've cleaned that kitchen today." Jon wears a look of disgust, shaking his head as he returns from downstairs with fresh water and chocolate-covered peanuts. "It's like all everyone does is run around eating, dirtying up dishes that I have to clean."

I try not to chortle. My belly rubs against the slanted lap-desk that straddles my middle. A wave of empathy crested with satisfaction ripples to my toes. "I'm sorry you had so much cleaning today."

"Are you laughing?" He halts halfway through pulling off his T-shirt. His clothes are wet with dishwater and his hair disheveled. He looks like he's been roughed up by our kitchen. "You're smiling."

"No. Really—" The laughter bursts from my throat. I can't hold it back.

He starts to chuckle. "So you think there's some sort of justice here? That this is my payback for years of never scraping my plate, for getting a fresh glass every time I had a drink of water?"

"I said nothing. Really . . . It's just that you call this a bad cleaning day. I call it Saturday."

"I'm certainly reformed after this." He finishes changing into pajamas and plops in bed. "What are you doing?"

Since my session with Dr. Geffen, I've sat with my stubborn fear and tried to stare it down, but my angst refuses to blink. For the times when my heart starts to race and I simply must look away, I've mastered the ultimate diversion: Internet shopping.

"Just picking up some holiday gifts." I look over at my closet, where three boxes that came today sit unopened. I examine Jon's face for traces of admonishment. "What do you think of this for Maddie?"

I show him the image of the lifelike doll, Baby Chou Chou.

"She cries when she's hungry or needs soothing, and sighs when she's content. Maddie can . . . you know . . . practice." The words feel awkward coming from my mouth, like I've just taken some liberty, crossed some treacherous line.

We take in the screen.

His eyes widen. "I'll set up the Pack 'N Play in her room. She can pretend to put her baby to sleep while we put our baby to sleep."

"And it says it comes with diapers. We can tell her she needs to practice with the doll before she can change the baby." I envision my imaginative daughter, meticulously applying the pretend ointment before snugly securing the diaper tabs on the pretend baby.

"I've heard horror stories about kids adjusting to new siblings. Maybe we can ease her into it, make it less hard on her."

Our faces light up, filled with visions of Maddie carrying her new baby alongside me carrying our new baby.

But what if we don't get a new baby?

I glimpse myself walking with empty arms beside my despondent daughter, clinging to the doll intended only as a precursor for our yearning, not a substitute.

My body stiffens. "Maybe this is a bad idea. I mean, if she constantly walks around with this doll, and something happens . . ."

The excitement trickles from Jon's face. We study the screen. He pulls my head to his shoulder, strokes my hair. "We wouldn't have to give it to her right away. We could wait. Until we're ready."

I look back toward the image, praying to see my daughter with this silly plastic toy.

⤳ DECEMBER 7

"Hi, I'm Gina." The exceptionally young ultrasound technician comes in and walks straight to the machine controls without looking at us. Her face looks grim, as if marked with long-standing disappointment. I look toward Jon. He shifts his eyes toward the table where I lie and grimaces.

"Have you ever had an ultrasound?" She snaps the sheath onto the probe.

My mouth drops. *Did she even glance at my chart?* "Many. Maybe a dozen with this pregnancy alone."

"Do you have any questions about the procedure?"

"No."

"Let's get started relax your legs while I insert the transducer." Her words spill out in one flat rush.

The probe burrows into my body. I jump. "Can you not press quite so hard?"

"The transducer needs to be fully inserted."

"I realize that. But it usually doesn't feel this uncomfortable." She eases up. A bit. I can't help but wonder about her work experience. There's a lot of art in taking correct cervical measurements, and as she fights my body and the machine, I question the depth of her experience.

In a key study that linked cervical length to the probability of early delivery, every technician who took measurements was specifically trained on how much pressure to apply to the cervix. If the technician applies too much pressure, the numbers are biased. The doctors who designed the study knew that operator error can affect results; they managed this potential pitfall.[19] As a patient, I need to manage it, too.

Gina holds the probe in place while pounding the wall to

summon Dr. Randolph. She moves to the corner and begins adjusting knobs on the ultrasound base while he mans the transducer. I watch as he repeats multiple measurements.

"Have you heard anything about the amnio?" Jon asks.

"No, not yet." Electronic Xs connected with a measured line appear on the screen before he asks Gina to leave and call about our amnio results.

"Dr. Randolph, I have to ask . . . I think Gina may be the sixth different ultrasound technician I've seen. Why do I always have a different technician?"

He looks at me, perplexed.

"I . . . I don't want to be offensive, but I know there's a lot of subjectivity with these measurements—not every technician does them the same. I'm worried that the numbers may not be reliable if there's a different person every time."

Dr. Randolph tightens his lip. He explains that he doesn't have a dedicated ultrasound technician for his office. "The hospital assigns a technician from a pool of possibilities each day. But you should note that I always confirm the measurement myself."

I now feel a little silly, realizing that this conscientious doctor does always recheck. My cheeks start to flush. He reviews the number for today: 26 millimeters.

"I am glad you brought it up. I would not want you going home worried about this." The corners of his mouth curl as he rests a hand on his hip.

~ ~ ~

Jon races to the ringing phone when we get back to the house. "He has the results?" Jon whips his head toward me.

I sit on the sofa. "Amnio?"

He nods. "I'm waiting for Dr. Randolph to come on."

I grab a pillow and clutch it to my stomach. *Please be good.* I don't know what we'd do if—

"I'm here." Jon's voice booms through the quiet room. He stiffens and listens.

Jon sighs. "It's okay. The amnio is normal," he says, covering the phone with his hand.

I throw the pillow aside and toss my feet up on the couch, snuggling under the thick, warm blanket. I slide down underneath and let my shoulders dissolve.

DECEMBER 8

"Okay, Maddie. We have a big surprise!" Jon doles out cupcakes around the tiny toddler table that now abuts the sofa for evening meals together. Maddie's face fills with the glee of delicious anticipation.

Jon visually checks me for final confirmation before spilling the news. "Remember when we told you that Mommy may have a baby in her tummy?"

Her face lights up and I chime in.

"We saw the doctor today, and now he's certain. There is a baby in my tummy."

"Yeah!" She screams and claps her hands.

I glance at Jon, knowing that we had to tell her something. I've been on bed rest for months and have gained twenty pounds—tangible proof of my pregnancy for her to see. She often eyes me suspiciously, and while she says nothing is on her mind, lately she hasn't wanted to go on play dates or to ballet, preferring to stay home with me. With the amnio results it feels like we should tell her, give her troubled mind some explanation for all of this. Still, I'm uncomfortable exposing her to a possibility that still looms with uncertainty.

"You're going to be a big sister this spring," Jon says.

She leaps from her chair. Jon and I wear painted smiles, but underneath we panic.

I've never been so torn at the sight of my daughter's joy. We all crave this baby—Maddie as much as Jon and me. But what will I tell her if we lose this baby? What if her ability to believe is forever diminished by another loss?

Maddie runs into the kitchen to grab milk for the cupcakes. I lean toward Jon and whisper, "Are we sure this was the right thing to do?"

He looks worried, but resolved. "Yes."

Maddie returns with three glasses and begins to pour milk from the carton. She now looks more subdued.

"Do you feel okay today, Mom?" She takes a sip and studies me with apprehension far beyond her years.

"I feel perfect, Maddie. Just perfect." I scrape the icing from the edges of the cupcake's paper wrapper. "Why do you ask?"

"No reason." She picks at the sprinkles atop the frosting.

"Maddie?" I look into her eyes. "Are you worried about the baby?"

Her expression becomes flat. She is silent.

"You know that I'm taking special medicine, so this baby will be okay."

"All Mommy needs to do is rest and take her medicine, and this baby will be fine." Jon strokes her cheek. "There's nothing to worry about."

"Daddy's right, sweetheart. This time is different. We know

the baby will be fine." My chest sinks, praying my words aren't exposed as a lie. And what if they are? What if her trust in us dissolves along with her ability to hope?

If only I didn't have to make these promises that may not be real, that I may not be able to control—but I've really no choice. Anything less than a complete assurance will leave her troubled and anxious for the months to come. I can't put that weight on her tender little shoulders.

Maddie nods a reluctant agreement.

"Hey, Miss girl. There's one last cupcake, and this is a special night. You could have two desserts. Do you want it?" I grin, knowing I've found her consistent delight.

She smiles appreciatively. "No thanks, Mom."

~ DECEMBER 9 *Nineteen weeks and five days*

My hand trembles. I'm not sure how long I've stared at the same page of jumpy words. Ten minutes? Twenty? I place the closed book on the nightstand, then pour the last glass of water from the pitcher where cubes have long melted.

Dr. Geffen was right; anniversary dates *are* agonizing. I didn't know this until a few years ago, having connected anniversaries with celebrations—weddings, birthdays—too inexperienced to know that loss also etches a date of remembrance.

I lost my twins on July Fourth. The date once brought wonder; lying outside in the dark, feasting on a night sky painted with impossible brilliance, bathing in the perfection of summer. I wonder if I'll ever feel the beauty, hear the booms without hope seeping from my sinking chest like a wounded balloon.

My twins were nineteen weeks and five days gestation when they died; the same exact age as this baby is today.

Think of Dr. Geffen's advice: when I can no longer face the fear, try distraction.

But what could possibly take my mind from this day in my last pregnancy, their last day?

Could they have been saved? If the doctor had done an ultrasound and measured my cervix the day before I lost them, when I went to the ER before my son's sac ruptured, could they have been saved?

If the doctor had considered that my mother had lost one baby in the second trimester and another in the third, if he'd tested for *inherited* thrombophilias after I'd lost two babies and not four, could my babies have been saved?

They would now be one-year-olds, if they were with me. Toddling through the house, taking first steps, walking on their toes instead of their feet. I wonder where they would walk to on those tiny toes? I wonder if they would laugh alike? Look alike?

I open the drawer of the nightstand and remove a thin black leather case shaped like an envelope, the slender case I carried on the plane from California, far too valuable to leave in the custody of movers. I open the flap and slide out the picture. Two little squiggles, side by side in matching sacs; life illustrated in the grainy image of an ultrasound. This image, the only one I have of them, when they were labeled Twin A and Twin B, before doctors would call them what they really were, my son, my daughter.

I hold the print at the edges, away from my face, careful to avoid damage from fingerprints or tears. I'm told the image will fade with time, and will disappear faster if exposed to heat and light. I keep it safe, in a black case, in a cool drawer, sometimes just touching the edges of the leather case, knowing what's inside. I can manage the heat and the light, but what about the time? What will be left when time drains the last proof of lives believed needlessly lost?

DECEMBER 16 *Twenty weeks and five days*

Maddie jumps from the chair when the doorbell chimes and then flings open the front door. Mary and her daughters stand outside, holding bags of takeout for dinner. She wears a long black coat stuffed with down, but miraculously maintains an hourglass outline.

"Guess what! Guess what!" She squeals. "There's a baby in my mommy's tummy!"

Mary starts to laugh, then feigns surprise. Maddie runs back to the sofa and rips the blanket down to my knees, revealing the proof of my bulging belly. Grace and Ally quickly follow and begin touching my stomach, inspecting the evidence.

"Why don't you ladies go play until I call you for dinner?" Mary sits in the leather chair and waits until the girls get up the stairs. "I see you told her."

"Yeah. And big-mouth is telling everyone. A few school parents have already called." I connected with these parents only briefly, during the first weeks of school before the bed rest. They called to express congratulations. Then they probed around the other part of Maddie's story, that Mommy had to lie down all the time. "I said something about lots of nausea. I can't really tell people what's going on."

"And what is going on? Have you seen any of your doctors this week?"

"I saw Dr. McConaughey a few days ago." I grab a cracker from the snack tray Mary centered on the coffee table. "But those visits aren't really exciting—no measurements or anything. We did talk about all the anxiety."

"Is it about something specific, or just the whole pregnancy?"

"Some of it's about my twins." I don't look at her. "This is around the time that I lost them, in the last pregnancy." I stiffen, returning for a moment to the ill-fated car ride to the hospital at midnight. I lay down in the backseat, watching the street lights flicker like strobes as Jon raced us to the hospital, already too late, already without hope. I'd been plagued by these memories in my sleep for weeks, but as the gestational anniversary of their deaths got closer, the flashbacks started to come throughout the day.

"I'm so sorry." She hugs me with a tight grasp, and I feel so lucky to know this glorious woman, knowing the value of such sincere friendship. We could have never recovered after losing our twins without the profound love of family and friends. I'll never forget how my girlfriends took time away from their jobs and their husbands and their children to be with me on Fridays, the day of the week when I lost them. For weeks I would break down every Friday at three-thirty, the time of his loss, feeling the horror as if it were happening all over again. My devoted friends cried with me and talked with me, and then one Friday, it was suddenly four-fifteen and I hadn't dissolved. If we weren't all now scattered in different cities, they would be with me now. Instead I hear their voices on regular phone calls and feel soothed by their familiar laughter; I also feel blessed with my new friend who feels as close as the women I've known for years.

"My therapist says that if I face the experience, feel the fear, the old hurt will be able to move through me. So that's what I've been trying to do, until I can't anymore."

"That sounds like good advice and all . . ." She walks over and props the pillow behind my head. "But right now, you're in the middle of a harrowing pregnancy. With all the problems, I can see how you'd be terrified. So it may not be so easy to sit with your fear until it goes away. That may not happen until you have your healthy baby."

"I think you may be right." I grab the last cracker from Mary's appetizer plate and stack it with the remnants of cheese. "That's why I'm turning to distraction. If it weren't for food and Internet shopping I think I'd go bonkers."

I crunch the tasty tidbit as Mary swipes the empty plate. She comes back from the kitchen with the platter stacked even higher than before.

∼ DECEMBER 18 *Twenty-one weeks*

"What should I do with these?"

The babysitter holds three cardboard boxes stacked atop one another. I glimpse the retailer names outside the boxes, but I've now bought so much online I can't remember what's inside each.

"Can you open them up and let me see what's there?"

The sitter, a stout immigrant taking odd jobs while on furlough, effortlessly rips the packaging tape with her hands.

The first contains more books to add to the growing stack by my bed. The next holds new basketball sneakers for Jon, a gift to encourage his Sunday night basketball league, a needed stress release.

"Ah! I know who this is for."

She holds up the baby doll that cries and sleeps, dressed in a pink sleeper, surrounded by miniature bottles and lotions and diapers.

"Should I wrap this for you?"

I hesitate. "No. Just put it in my closet. On the top shelf."

DECEMBER 23 *Twenty-one weeks and five days*

"I don't feel well." I press my back into our headboard as Jon's sleepy eyes widen. "I don't think it's the baby," I quickly add. "I just feel woozy."

He slides his hand across my forehead and then walks to the medicine cabinet for a thermometer. After shaking down the ancient mercury-filled tube, he holds it up to the morning light before placing it under my tongue.

"Is Mommy sick?" Maddie stumbles into our bedroom rubbing her eyes, dragging her animal blanket behind her. She's suddenly more alert.

"I'm fine, sweetheart. Did you sleep well?" My words are choppy, choked by the stick gripped between my teeth. She nods and crawls into my bed, studying me before grabbing the TiVo remote to start an *Arthur*. Before she finds the episode, I bolt from the bed toward the bathroom. I'm within arm's length of the toilet when green vomit spews.

"Dad! Come quick!" Maddie runs after me, her five-year-old eyes alarmed. She wets a washcloth and brings it to me. "Is the baby okay?"

"The baby is fine. Mommy's just a little sick." Jon leans down to speak to her and pushes a thick red curl behind her ear.

"I'm a little sick, Maddie, but nothing that could hurt a baby." I try to sound convincing and casual.

Jon scans the bathroom, surveying the mess.

"I'm sorry, but I couldn't make it—" My body heaves and I throw up some more. When I'm sure there can't possibly be anything left, the rest comes. Bitter. "It's probably just a bug. Awful, but likely nothing." I wipe my mouth with the wet cloth.

"I'll help you change."

Jon takes my arm to help me up. When I lift my head, the room spins. "Oh. No. Can't go anywhere yet. Too dizzy." I retreat back to the bathroom floor. Sharp pains grip my stomach.

~ ~ ~

"Your labs are back. Your white blood count is elevated." Dr. Berkeley, the same ER doc that I saw in October, walks to the machine that records contractions and fetal heartbeat and looks at the graphed scroll it spits out. "The fetal heart rate is regular and strong. That's a good sign."

I nod, grateful for her assurance, but still unsettled.

"Are you still cramping?"

"Yes, but it feels mild. Is the machine picking up any sort of pattern?"

"It's not recording any contractions, but these monitors often fail to pick them up before twenty-four weeks." She checks the IV bag, nearly drained. "You also show signs of dehydration."

"She always gets dehydrated." Jon sits in a stiff recliner in the corner, slouching as though his body is being drained into a spout. Maddie lies by his feet on the floor, pretending to color while she listens to every word. "That's why I made her come in," he says to the doctor.

"I've only needed IV fluids a few times in the twelve years

that I've known this man." I rise up on my elbows and shoot Jon a look of playful annoyance, trying to bait my husband into banter that may distract him, make him seem less spent.

"Your cramping may be the result of dehydration. Let's pump you full of fluids and keep monitoring for a few hours."

"Do you think it's preterm labor?" Jon asks.

"Let's keep an eye on her and see if the cramping subsides. But no, at this point, the most likely explanation is a virus, maybe something gastrointestinal."

"I wasn't sure what to think. With the vomiting, then the cramping . . ." I press against the uterine monitor, a device that resembles an air hockey paddle threaded through a wide elastic band, and hold it closer to my stomach.

"You did the right thing by coming in." Dr. Berkeley squeezes my hand. "You need to make sure."

DECEMBER 24 *Twenty-one weeks and six days*

"I haven't felt quite right since yesterday." I wedge my ankles into the stirrups while Dr. Randolph begins the examination.

"She was dehydrated. I think they gave her three bags of fluid before we left." Today Jon stands by the head of the exam table.

Dr. Randolph intensely studies the ultrasound screen. When I called to tell him about the ER visit yesterday, he asked me to come in immediately. None of the technicians began today's exam. He's done everything himself.

His solemn expression betrays some concern.

"What's the cervical measurement?" Jon asks.

Dr. Randolph moistens his lips, keeps them open a moment

before responding. "It is relatively stable—twenty-four millimeters, so not much change from the last measurement. But if you look here"—he points to a dark spot on the image projected onto the screen—"there is some funneling."

My chest sinks. Funneling has been associated with preterm labor, an additional signal that my baby is at higher risk. The frozen image on the screen looks as though the inside of the cervix has begun to open, and the sac has drooped toward the birth canal.

"This is the first time we have seen any funneling. It is a small amount, but noteworthy."

Jon steps closer as Dr. Randolph explains what funneling means.

"If the inside of the cervix continues to open, the funnel could descend so far as to meet the cerclage." Dr. Randolph studies the image as though he's sizing it up. "But it doesn't often progress that far. And if it does, that is what the cerclage is there for—to provide a barrier to retain the membranes, if necessary."

"Will the cerclage hold, if the funnel does go that low?" I lift my head to see the doctor's face, try to deduce any emotion that may cling to his detached words.

"That is the key question." Dr. Randolph folds his arms, raises his chin. "We expect that it should." He pauses, then interprets our silence as his cue to leave the room.

Jon hands me my shirt as I push away the crinkling paper sheet and sit up. I feel anxious, tense; agitated that yet another peril has been added to our already full plate. I examine Jon's face for his reaction, wondering if he feels any fear, and if he doesn't, whether he'll be able to understand mine.

The old scripts play through my mind from years ago, when he smirked at my caution and marginalized my worry. I hear his old words in his old voice—the one before our last loss—and I listen for a moment before the sounds grow silent, leaving my fists clenched.

"Let's not say anything. Let's just use your scale. What do you think, on a scale of one to ten?" I wait for his response.

He lowers his head, casts his eyes toward the ground. "Four."

My chest loosens. I close my eyes and listen again to the word just spoken. *Four. He thinks it's a four.*

I take soothing breaths as I slide on my maternity jeans. "Then we're in the same place today." I take my husband's hand and hold it as we walk to the elevator.

DECEMBER 27 *Twenty-two weeks and two days*

"Do you want to light the candles?" Jon strikes a match and ignites the Shamash, held firmly in Maddie's fingers. We recite the blessing as she passes the flame across all eight Hanukkah candles, her face bathed in a growing glow.

"Did you get more gelt, Daddy?" Maddie clasps her expectant hands.

Jon puffs his chest and empties pockets filled with chocolate coins, glistening in their golden wrappers. "These are the ones from the candy maker around the corner, like we had on Tuesday." Jon stacks the candy in tall towers while Maddie spins the crystal dreidel, her gift the first night of Hanukkah.

"Gimel!" She takes the two pieces of gelt on the table, prying off the wrappers and tossing the chocolate into her mouth. Between turns she glances toward the dining room table where two wrapped packages wait. She doesn't know that upstairs, pushed back on the top shelf of my closet, there's a third—the doll that cries and laughs, demands to be cared for—her practice doll for learning to care for her new sibling.

I stretch my arm across the table pushed against the sofa and spin the dreidel. "Gimel for me, too." I follow her lead and gobble my bounty.

"Mom?" She eyes me curiously. "When you eat the gelt, is the baby getting some, too?"

Jon smiles. "Sure. Sure. The baby gets some of whatever Mommy eats."

"How?"

I say something about a cord that's like a straw. She looks puzzled.

"But how did the straw get in there? And how did the baby get there?"

"Is it time for presents?" Jon asks.

She leaps from the chair and runs to the dining room, shredding the paper on the biggest box within seconds. She hugs the neck of the stuffed dog sent from Nanny and Poppop. Then she mauls the second, eyes wide when the pink Barbie Jeep from my sister emerges from the tattered paper.

Jon catches my eye while she packs the Jeep with Barbies. He silently mouths *"Doll?"* and throws his head toward the stairs.

I look toward the menorah, where the last of our candles are nearly extinguished. I want to give it to her, but I run my hand across my belly, still unsettled, crampy for days now. I look toward Jon and shake my head helplessly.

He nods before sitting on the floor to play Barbie with Maddie.

DECEMBER 30 *Twenty-two weeks and five days*

I open my eyelids. Heavy. Can't believe this is real. Can't comprehend what just happened. My little boy, my precious little boy. Did I really just lose him? Did I really just push my son into a world that offered him only death?

Have to protect her. Keep her safe. Hold my cupped hand against my belly.

Dr. D stands with his surgical mask pulled below his chin. He studies the floor, as does a nurse. Jon sits in a chair in the corner. His eyes are closed, his mouth held as though grasping horror with his teeth.

The bleeps of the heart rate monitors echo through the room. Two bleeps. I watch the white lines roll across the machine, watch the numbers change.

The nurse steps out of the room, glances toward me from the doorway. Quickly looks away when I look back.

Dr. D picks up a chart from the table piled with sheets and towels. The paper on the clipboard crinkles when he lifts the page.

I look at the clouds barely visible through the cracked blinds. Weak light filters through. I wonder if they could open the window?

The IV drips. One drop. Then another. It looks wet. Water. I'd like some water.

My head swims. I push back the blankets and caress my belly. Look toward Jon in the chair. His face no longer contorted. Flat. Eyes still closed. Grasping the arms of the chair.

I run my hand across my head, wipe away beads of sweat. Hot sweat.

I am hot.

I am hot.

I look toward Dr. D. Does he suspect?

Pull the blanket back over my shoulders. Protect her. Can't fail her. Turn on my side, away from his clinical eyes.

I watch her heart rate. 156. 152. 152.

This will pass. Can't let them know.

Close my eyes. Drift.

I see them. My beautiful babies. They sit, looking at one another with huge soft eyes of the purest blue, and faces filled with amazement. Tufts of fair hair cover little rounded heads and frame tiny pink ears. I need to hold them, touch them, run my finger across their soft round cheeks. I try to get closer, but I'm stuck. I struggle, resist. I can't get to them.

Eyes open. Jon looks at me, reddened eyes full.

My poor husband. Such sadness. I push the blankets off my chest. Need to cool off. Turn my head. Hold my belly. Start to float.

I see them again. My babies coo. They reach their hands out toward one another. Such love with twins. Such connection.

I look closer. What do they look like? Do they have my eyes, or Jon's chin, like Maddie? Do they look like Maddie?

Maddie. My blessed daughter. How I love her. I see her now.

She turns toward me. Her red hair is held tight from her face and her crystal blue eyes are filled with tears. Her fair face drips with sadness.

Why is she so sad? Maddie? Maddie!

I toss my head. Try to call her name.

Why is my little girl crying?

Maddie!

"Hot."

The word slips from my lips. I open my eyes. Dr. D tilts his head toward me.

"What? What did you say, Darci?"

He inspects me.

"Get a temperature. Now."

My God! What did I do? I have to protect my baby. What have I just done?

The nurse pulls the standing thermometer closer. Jabs the stick under my tongue. Beep. "102."

Dr. D says something to the nurse. She runs out. Jon springs from the chair.

"Darci. We need to take this baby." The doctor grips the rails of my bed, leans closer to my face.

I turn away. Close my eyes. This isn't real.

"Darci. You must listen. You have a fever. I suspect infection."

I throw the blankets back. "Hot. Need some water." I rise toward the water pitcher. I'll get her some water. Fall back toward the bed. Close my eyes.

"Darci. We need to take the baby. I need your permission." His insistent tone stings my ears and his breath rolls in blusters across my face.

I raise my trembling hand, try to push him away. This isn't real. I had to let him go, my precious little boy. So brave, going to save your sister.

"Do it. My God! Take the baby," Jon shouts.

Footsteps. Hurried. Must be running, scurrying around the bed.

"I need permission from Darci."

"I am giving you permission. Look at her. Take the baby!"

"I CAN'T. Not without her permission. Darci. DARCI!" the doctor screams, not allowing the escape of unconsciousness again.

"NO. She is fine." My eyes fly open. I look at her heartbeat. 150. 152. Glare back at the doctor. We let him go to save her. We're supposed to save her.

"We have to take her. If we wait, antibiotics may not work. There may be nothing I can do for you. Infection can quickly get out of control. We have to take her. NOW."

"No! Please! God, no." I can't let her go my God I can't my baby my baby this isn't supposed to happen I won't lose them both toss my head Drip Beep Run Push.

"I can't lose her. Please! Please, Dr. D!"

"I'm sorry. I am so sorry, but we need your permission. Please. PLEASE Let Me Take Her."

"Tell him yes! Darci! Tell Him YES!" Jon pleads.

Nurses scatter Jon pulls the top of his hair with clenched hands no God no.

Maddie's soulless face.

"Darci!" Jon screams.

Oh! God! I love you my little angel. I love you. How can I give them permission to take you?

Toss my head. Close my eyes tighter.

"DARCI!" Jon screams and pleads.

I'm so sorry little girl they said we could save you I said I'd protect you God why can't I protect her I tried I tried.

I cover my face and scream.

Please forgive me I'm so sorry please forgive me God why can't I protect my tiny princess please forgive me Mommy tried Mommy tried. Oh God.

". . . temp is rising . . ."

"DARCI."

Drifting. No. Please.

I quake as though shaking out the word that must be said.

"Yes."

Dr. D pulls the mask over his nose, black eyes bulging through the sliver of skin separating his mask and cap.

I wail a deep, bottomless cry. Nurses hold my bent legs as the doctor grabs a slender pointed rod from the tray. Warm liquid fills the bed.

"No! God NO!" I scream. Jon clasps my shaking hand, lets out a deep moan.

I feel her. Slipping. Faster. I can't let her go. How can I stop it? I can't I can't I have to let her go. God! She slides farther and I can't *turn her away can't fail her not look at her as though she's to be abhorred I'm so sorry thrust forward please forgive me try and see her just once before my angel goes away.*

The world goes black.

JANUARY

"Jon. Jon!" I shake my husband in the dark room.

"Huh. HUH?" He jumps, sitting upright in bed.

"I need you to get up. We need to go to the hospital."

He rushes to his closet. "Are you cramping?"

"Yes. And now there's back pain."

"What should we do with Maddie?"

"We can't wake up a neighbor at five o'clock. We'll have to take her."

We carry our sleepy daughter to the car and are gone within minutes.

~ ~ ~

"When did the cramping start?" The same ER doc from a few weeks ago tightens the fetal monitoring strap across my stomach.

"It's been a while. I don't think it ever went away completely, after the virus last week."

"Are you familiar with the pain rating scale?" She references a poster depicting a series of simple drawings, starting with a contented face at 0 and ending with the tortured expression of a 10.

"It's mild, but there's a constant discomfort. Maybe on the scale it's a four."

Jon listens from the chair where Maddie rests on him, still in her pajamas, half asleep.

"My biggest concern is the back pain. That's why I came in." The pain radiates down my lower back. I know this pain, the message it sends. "I've only had this type of pain when I was in labor, or miscarrying."

The throb and pulse of these rhythmic pangs were etched in my mind the last time I had them—when I lost my twins. I am only twenty-three weeks, just outside any chance of viability for my baby. If the baby comes now, there will be nothing they can do. Another precious little baby will—

Deep breath. Feel the air as it fills my lungs. Breathe.

I close my eyes and clench the sheets in closed fists, forcing air deep into my chest. *Calm.* This is different. I'm at the hospital, getting every possible treatment this time. I focus on the sounds in the room: the doctor's footsteps, the chair that squeaks beneath Jon and Maddie, the regular beeps that bring proof of our baby's steady heartbeat.

"Can you bend your legs?" The doctor sits on a round stool and explains that she needs to do a noninvasive vaginal examination. "I don't want to risk inserting a speculum if you're already unsteady, but I do need to look for emergent signs of labor."

"Jon, can you take Maddie out?" She watches from the chair, her eyes no longer filled with sleep, but apprehension. A nurse offers to take her for juice and graham crackers. I look toward Jon.

"I should take her." He clasps her hand and leads her toward the door.

"Sweetheart?" Maddie stops and looks. "Mommy is fine, and so is the baby. The doctor just needs to check something, okay?"

Maddie nods, but doesn't speak. I hear Jon ask her if she's worried as they enter the hall. "I'm ready now." I obediently bend my legs.

The doctor pulls an overhead light closer, turns it on. The glare makes me squint. "No visible membranes." She presses, lifts. My legs warm from the beam before she turns it off and stands. "There are no signs of dilation."

Dr. Berkeley grabs the scrolled tape from the contraction monitor, running her eyes over the lines. "It's not picking up anything."

What does she mean by that? I think back to my twins, when I went to the ER knowing something was wrong, accepting their false reassurances over my own intuition, and returning just twelve hours later with the bitter proof of their miscalculation. I won't let it happen to this baby.

I catch her eye. "Dr. Berkeley, regardless of what the monitor shows, this pain is very real."

"I believe you," she says without hesitation.

~ ~ ~

"This back pain just isn't normal, Dr. Randolph. I know that something's not right, regardless of what the contraction monitor said."

Jon and I sit with Dr. Randolph in his conference room, grateful that Mary came and picked up Maddie hours ago. After four hours of monitoring in the ER, the machine found no proof of my pain; the device often cannot detect contractions before twenty-four weeks. The attending physician called Dr. Randolph before ordering my discharge, and he asked me to come see him immediately.

"Your cervix has not changed from the last exam." Dr. Randolph looks at his notes from my visit last week. "You were twenty-six millimeters today, so the number appears stable."

"What about the funneling? Is that more of a concern, given her pain?" Jon asks.

"The funneling has not progressed since last week."

"Then what do you think is going on? Why am I having these symptoms?"

"Well, some of your symptoms are consistent with preterm labor." He pauses, juts out his chin. "On the other hand, we have objective measures that indicate stability with a week ago." His face is calm, relaxed. "Let's not lose sight of that."

"So what do we do?" I unfold the discharge instructions on the table. The paper says I should stay on complete bed rest, getting up only to go to the bathroom, and lie on my left side to maximize fetal blood flow. "I've already been doing this. Is there anything else?" I throw up my hands. "Should I be on medication to fend off the contractions?"

He looks skeptical.

"I realize the machine isn't picking anything up, but Dr. Randolph, I feel them in my back. They are very real."

"There are medications used to manage contractions, but we do not prescribe them before twenty-four weeks," he responds. "It's not thought safe before then."

I nod. I won't do anything that's not safe for my baby, but exactly what is the safe option, that one that assures me a healthy, term baby? "How about steroids? Should we do steroid injections to speed lung development?"

The most common cause of preterm fatalities is respiratory distress syndrome. Most babies don't reach full lung development until around thirty-two weeks. Steroid injections delivered in utero can speed lung development, diminishing the most common threat to premature babies. Maddie had one injection, twelve hours before she was born; the treatment requires two injections administered over forty-eight hours to reach full effectiveness. When she came at only twenty-eight weeks, after just hours of treatment, her lungs weren't fully developed, and she struggled against respiratory distress syndrome. I still remember the hiss of the ventilator each time the accordion chamber compressed, forcing air into her helpless little lungs.

"Steroids are not used prior to twenty-four weeks. There are risks from the treatment, and the earlier the injections, the higher the risk to the baby." He looks stern. "The treatment does speed lung development, but I would only recommend steroids as a last resort, if we thought the chance of early delivery was extremely high."

My heart pounds. I'd tucked away the option of steroids in my mind like a huge cushion for my baby. Even though Maddie had just a few hours of treatment, the doctors believed it was a likely savior for her. I never thought about the possible risk of the treatment, never realized that this safety net had holes.

"Darci, this is not something we need to think about right now. Indications are stable. Labor does not appear imminent." He casts a look of reassurance and concern.

I sit back, wanting to believe, but the pain that still radiates down my back speaks loudly, accompanied by the searing knowledge of past false hope, when only I knew something was wrong.

I glance toward Jon, and he looks less resolute than this

morning, more at ease. Was the angst he felt hours ago quelled by the stock reassurances of the doctors and the machines? And if it was, will he understand why my symptoms and my intuition supercede their removed speculation?

"We'll have you back in a few days, just before twenty-four weeks, to check for indications of preterm labor. In the meantime, go back home. Get in bed." Dr. Randolph pauses. "And if the pain gets worse, you can come back. Immediately."

JANUARY 4 *Twenty-three weeks and three days*

"Your friend is here." Our babysitter, the fourth so far, stands in my bedroom, holding folded laundry for the closets.

"Can you ask her to come up?"

Since the last doctor's appointment, I have left my bed only to go to the bathroom. My lower back still throbs. Dull. Constant. Regardless of what the monitors pick up, what the measurements indicate, I know that my pregnancy is in jeopardy. I *feel* it. If I can just lie still, make it a few more days, this baby will have some chance of survival; at twenty-four weeks, 40 percent of preemies survive. At this point, every day I sustain this pregnancy makes a critical difference.

Mary walks into my room carrying a handful of magazines. I'm trying to look brave, but as her expression dissolves, I know I haven't pulled it off. I slide up on the pillows and try to steady myself with short breaths.

"Are you still worried?"

I nod. If I speak, I might weep.

"It's okay." She pulls up the chair Jon carried in from the dining room. "You still have the back pain?"

My eyes start to fill.

She folds her arms and scans the room before grabbing the empty pitcher on my nightstand and returning with ice water.

"How's Jon doing with all of this?" She pours a glass of water for each of us.

"I think he's worried. But it seems . . . different for him."

Jon's life is hell right now. We have some babysitting to help with Maddie, but he still needs to go to work and then come home to endless tasks. He rarely has a moment to himself. I know he's worried, but I feel like his hell is mostly about over-work, not the kind of pervasive panic that often keeps me up at night, or brings nightmares when sleep does come.

"He is supporting me. He's taking care of us, and he doesn't question my decisions anymore." I run my finger along the edge of the water glass. "But to be honest, I'm having trouble letting go of the other pregnancies, when he didn't get it."

We talk about the visits with Dr. Randolph, when I hear news that makes me quiver. Jon doesn't challenge my reaction, but most of the time, he seems unaffected. "Maybe he doesn't react because he doesn't understand all the medical stuff, and I can't really be upset about that. He hasn't studied it, and he seems to respect that I have—I feel like he trusts my decisions."

"That's so important. It feels awful to be second-guessed."

I nod, thinking about how I'm always waiting for one of our old fights to explode. And it's not really fair of me. He's been great during this pregnancy. "I just need to let go of all of our old crap, leave it in the past."

"Sometimes that's hard to do. Especially if you're scared that the past might be repeated."

"I know. But I should. I can see that it's different for him now." And how could it not be, with everything we've been through? I look down at the blanket and fiddle with the edges.

"You know the other thing?" I lean toward Mary. "I feel awful for saying this, but . . . if I lose this baby, I don't know what it will do to my marriage." Now I start to cry.

For twelve years Jon and I have shared a solid connection that has never dissolved, even as tragedy wedged between us. When he couldn't understand what I was going through, we could still sit down together, talk, and immediately connect to that part of ourselves where love is unquestionable, unyielding, even when not all-knowing. But despite the strength of our bond, a part of me can't forget the pain when he didn't understand why I had to keep grieving after my losses, especially the months when I continued to grieve the loss of our twins, when my spirit couldn't return.

I know that we both felt their loss. He arranged a vacation immediately, got us all away from the house filled with anguish, and he took care of me when I cried, and sometimes cried with me. But as weeks of grief turned to months, I felt the subtleties of his impatience—exasperated sighs, stern glances, hurried conversations. I began to feel his judgment instead of his compassion, and a tension grew between us that only recently began to diminish.

"You're not going to lose this baby." Mary looks confident. "Look how vigilant you are, and you're getting treatment." She sits down on my bed. "Sometimes when we want something, we need to see it in our minds. I think you need to visualize yourself, with the baby, healthy."

"I try. I want to believe . . . I do. I'm just so scared."

"I want you to think about you and the baby, and Jon. You need to see how happy you all are."

I close my eyes and try to see myself holding this baby, staring into my husband's eyes, past hurts finally laid to rest.

"The first step to making anything true is to believe. You have to see it, and let yourself believe." Mary clasps her hand atop mine, and we sit in silence, filling the room with our visions.

JANUARY 6 *Twenty-three weeks and five days*

"Did you notice the fresh arugula and roasted red peppers?" Jon sits in the tiny toddler chair next to Maddie's play table that's now our permanent dining spot. He takes a break from his work to have lunch with me, making gourmet sandwiches to quell my appetite and my anxiety.

I lean on my side to eat from the plate placed on the bed, pushing a pillow next to the heating pad against my back. "It's delicious. A really nice touch."

"What have you done this morning?"

"I did the grocery shopping. It's set for delivery tomorrow afternoon." I take another bite of the sandwich, wondering what women did on bed rest before the Internet.

"Did you get milk?"

"Of course. Do you think I'd let my girl run out of milk?"

He starts to speak, then stops.

"What?"

"Well, it's just that, we have four gallons of milk already."

"Oh. I didn't know. I mean, I haven't been to the refrigerator in weeks."

"It's okay. Maybe you could order some pudding mix next time."

I nod at his accommodating suggestion. Over the past few days Jon has been exceptionally attentive, sometimes making my lunch himself instead of asking the babysitter to do it, and taking a few minutes to just sit with me. Still, I worry that he will tire of my anxiety and my inability to embrace the doctors who say that my pregnancy is stable, that I just need to stay on bed rest. I try to take Mary's suggestion and visualize us together, happy, with the new baby, but my memory instead turns to one of the old fights when he chided me for not trusting the doctor, and the sear of past words suddenly becomes fresh.

"So, do you think I'm being ridiculous, staying in our bedroom, not even going downstairs to the couch?"

"No. We agreed. Anything you need to do."

I take one of the carrot sticks from my plate and rise up on my elbow. "You know that doctors don't have all the answers, here—that OBs have to make a ton of judgment calls because there's so little solid research about pregnancy loss."

The causes of miscarriage are largely unexplored because obstetric research is grossly underfunded. In a neglected medical science like obstetrics, doctors often rely on the will of patients to keep trying, loss after loss, as though it's acceptable for women to lose children today simply because they can try again tomorrow; as though the individual babies lost have no inherent value.

I've already lost four children, and my body tells me that I may be about to lose a fifth. How much blind faith can I have in a science that relies on resilience as much as research?

I steady myself and ease back under the comforter. "Jon, I'm not trying to be difficult. It's just that I really need to feel your full support this time. And I don't believe we can have complete faith in what the doctors say." I shake my head. "With the twins, they didn't know. When I knew something was wrong and we went to the hospital, they sent us home. And we lost them the very next day. Look what our belief cost us."

Jon releases a deflated breath. "I get it. Darci, I do." he says. "We've been through so much, with the miscarriages, and then the twins."

He sits on the bottom of our bed. "I have to be honest. The first two miscarriages, they didn't mean that much to me. It's not that I didn't want the babies, but it just happened so early, it was like they were never real."

The grip of my chest starts to loosen. We've talked about the losses before, but Jon has never said what it really meant to him. I sit up.

"Then there were the twins." He shakes his head. "They were people, tiny little people, as big as some of the babies we saw in the NICU."

He covers his eyes.

I lean forward and rub his shoulder.

"They would have been one now. We would have had a couple of babies running around the house right now." He looks over at me. "Do you ever think about that?"

"Yes. I think about it all the time." I never knew he thought about it, too.

My heart breaks for my husband, seeing the pain in his face, intimately understanding the anguish I never knew he still felt. The past resentments and slights dissolve before me as I sit with my husband, inside as shaken by all we've lost as I am.

"I'm sorry for your pain. And I understand it, you know." I lean close and put my head on his shoulder.

He nods, squeezes my hand.

"So I do get it now, and I agree that we need to take every precaution to protect this baby."

"I'm so glad we're talking. I've been worried that you might be questioning whether all of this is necessary." I clutch my arms to my chest. "When we see Dr. Randolph, he says things that terrify me, and, it's like, well—you don't respond. I get scared that you won't support me."

I feel foolish. I've read so much into Jon's responses, as though there's only one legitimate way to react to our situation. I realize I haven't given my husband the latitude he needed to deal with our hardship in his own way, without the harshness of my judgment, my skepticism—the acceptance I've craved from him. In this latest phase of our long-standing struggle, I've nursed past hurts instead of welcoming a more understanding reality.

He shrugs his shoulders. "I do support you. And we're going to listen to what your body says this time."

He rises and starts to take my empty plate from the bed. "I believe it's the right thing to do."

I grab his hand, rub it against my cheek.

JANUARY 7 *Twenty-three weeks and six days*

Dr. Randolph knocks before coming in. He doesn't rush to his usual position, but stands close, where I can see his eyes. Calm. Nonjudgmental. He asks about the symptoms from last week.

"Dr. Randolph, my back still throbs, and my stomach feels tight."

"She hasn't been up for anything. She's been flat in bed since last week," Jon adds.

Dr. Randolph pauses before walking to the end of the table, claiming his usual prop from the technician. His assistant leans against a wall and stares at the images with wide eyes as Dr. Randolph maneuvers the probe. We all watch the shadowy monitor as if it were a crystal ball.

Relax my muscles. Relax. I close my eyes and will my pelvic muscles to ease, ignoring the foreign instrument that prods and presses. *Relax.* These measurements have to be right; they feel especially important today, as my back throbs, my stomach knots. I exhale and look toward Dr. Randolph as he measures the electronic line segments. He says nothing as more lines are drawn. Then more. His forehead puckers. My heart starts to sink.

"It appears . . . that there has been significant cervical shortening since your last visit. You are down to fourteen millimeters."

My chest burns. At 14 millimeters, research found that 30 to 50 percent of women will deliver preterm[20,21]; these studies were based on the general population of women, not "high-risk" women. With my history of late loss, my risk can only be worse.

"What about the funneling?" Jon sits up.

"The funnel has progressed. It now reaches the cerclage." An exasperated breath slips from his lips as he leans against the exam table.

I try to stay calm, but my breaths are becoming short and rapid. The funnel means that my baby's sac is dropping toward the birth canal, a warning sign in addition to the cervical measurement. Research predicts that more than half of all pregnancies will suffer premature rupture of the fetal membranes when funneling reaches the level of the cerclage.[22] This degree of funneling is dire.

Cervical incompetence often presents as ruptured membranes, and I know all too well what happens when the fetal sac tears; it was the rupture of my twin son's sac that signaled the end of his life, and the life of his sister. I went to the bathroom and saw my sanitary pad soaked from clear fluid flecked with dark little specs. It was amniotic fluid, leaking from my son's torn sac.

I look toward Dr. Randolph, open my mouth, but no words come out. His face is marked with alarm. Then he rights himself, staring back at the still image on the monitor.

"We need to administer steroid injections." Dr. Randolph stares intently. "We should do them tomorrow."

Just five days ago, despite my cramping and back pain and insistence that something was wrong, Dr. Randolph thought we wouldn't need the medication, thought that my chance of preterm labor wasn't high enough to risk these injections. Now my cervix has rapidly shortened, and the funnel has progressed down to the cerclage—objective proof of the truth only I knew—and now he believes me, now he is convinced that something is wrong.

I am terrified of my newfound credibility.

"What about the risk from the injections?" I remember his warning of the risk just days ago.

"There are risks from steroid injections. But I'm more concerned about the risk of preterm delivery at this point. I have seen patients who delivered at twenty-four weeks, without the steroids." He looks shaken. "You do not want to be in that position. The prognosis for the baby would be extremely poor."

My head starts to swim. "Can we do the injections today?"

"No. We need to wait until twenty-four weeks. We can't administer the first injection before tomorrow."

My God. He thinks I may lose this baby.

I try to turn my thoughts, but they scurry too quickly in opposite, dark directions.

Forty percent survival rate at twenty-four weeks.

I am not in labor at this moment; my baby is safe, at this moment. *Stay in this moment. Don't let the fear overtake me.*

I look toward Jon and feel my horror contorting my face. He leans toward me with a placid expression. As he reads me, concern descends over him like a revelation.

My eyes dart to the corners of the room across the panels of lowered ceiling and recessed lights and my fear begins screaming ominous predictions in my head.

Months in an NICU, if the baby survives.

I am getting treatment. This time can be different.

High chance of lifetime disabilities, if the baby survives.

We're watching everything. If I go into labor—

Sixty percent fatalities.

~ ~ ~

"How are you?" Ev asks.

"I . . . I'm . . . not really very good." I start to cry. My mother-in-law has called me almost every day of this pregnancy. Even on the tougher days, I stay upbeat, savoring our phone calls, using them to connect to the carefree nature of the past decade we've spent together. When she and Steve visit, they dote over Maddie, fill the house with fresh food and flowers, and slap a glass of wine in my hand the moment I'm home from work. My connection to them has always been about the joy in life; today, there is only intense fear.

"What's wrong? Did something happen?"

I've never once called her up in tears. I speak in whimpers instead of words.

"Take a deep breath." She waits, and when I can't quite pull myself together, I hear her faint gulps, no doubt swallowing her own tears.

"The doctor wants me to get steroid injections tomorrow. He thinks we may need them." I tell her about the measure-

ments, the funneling that now reaches the cerclage, the screaming back pain, and about the drugs thought too risky just days
earlier.

"What am I going to do? If my baby comes now, this child
may not even survive." I can't lose another baby. The pain of
losing my children still darkens my mind, leaves me crushed
beneath the weight of hopeless desire. I don't know if I can re-
cover again.

After the last loss I cried for months. It was all I could do to
contain my anguish until Maddie was at preschool. I poured
myself out to my therapist twice a week, desperate to reconnect
with my extinguished self, fighting to remember what the world
looked like in color.

I went to a celebration at Maddie's preschool for Sukkot, a
holiday about trusting in God's abundance. The children laughed
and sang and ate, and as I looked at their gleeful faces under the
sukkah, I could only stare at my watch and count the hours until
I could go to bed that night.

Other days I was overwhelmed with panic, gripped with fear
that Maddie wasn't safe. I would race to her preschool hours before dismissal, yielding to the tortuous conclusion that tragedy
was pervasive; that she was safe only if she was with me. It took
every ounce of self-control I had to sign her out at the office
instead of bursting through the classroom door to sweep her
into my arms.

"And Maddie. My God! She knows. We had to tell her.
How will she deal with another loss?" I weep at the thought
of my kindergartner, again facing the cruelty and senselessness
of death. If this baby dies, how will she reconcile the com-
plexities of a world where loss leaves even the edges of joy
elusive?

"We're coming for a visit. When Steve gets home, we'll figure out when we can come."

~ JANUARY 8 *Twenty-four weeks*

"Do you want this in the hip or the thigh?" The nurse holds a long needle just pulled from a vacuumed package.

I brace myself against the hospital recliner, enclosed by the curtain that nonetheless reveals a sliver of the other partially shrouded patient.

"My hips can't take any more shots." I push down my sweat pants, exposing hips that are mottled masses of purples and greens.

The nurse jumps before composing herself, then glances at my paperwork on her clipboard. "Heparin?"

I nod. "How about my butt? I can't reach there myself. You wouldn't be using any space I'll need."

She opens a towelette infused with alcohol.

I am twenty-four weeks pregnant. Twenty-four weeks.

I have seen the struggle of babies born at twenty-four weeks. When Maddie was in the NICU, I remember the tiny baby boy who came sixteen weeks too early. A delicate poster reading "Baby Boy Lowe" hung on the outside of his incubator. All the babies had these posters, most without a first name, at least for the first few days, when parents were still shocked, unprepared for what wasn't expected. Baby Boy Lowe weighed less than a pound, less than a package of butter. His blushed body was wrapped in a clear plastic suit, lying idle under the warmth of a glaring light that gave heat to this baby with no outermost layer of skin and no ability to regulate his own temperature.

When Maddie was born at twenty-eight weeks she weighed more than three pounds. Her tiny body looked enormous against so many of the other NICU babies. The doctors said she was huge for her gestational age, that she might have been ten pounds if she'd made it to full term. They believed that her substantial weight was a fundamental reason why she overcame the perils of prematurity. Smaller preemies have a worse prognosis than larger ones.

The nurse slips the needle into my skin. I don't jump, still not immune to the stab, but somehow numb.

Forty percent survival rate at twenty-four weeks.

"All done," she says, pressing a cotton pad against the puncture. "And you need to be back at the same time tomorrow for the second injection. It's important that the second shot be given twenty-four hours after the first."

"I'll be back tomorrow, at exactly one o'clock." I pull up my sweats and gather my purse, still thinking about the little boy who still lived in the NICU when Maddie came home.

I wonder what happened to Baby Boy Lowe?

✒ JANUARY 10 *Twenty-four weeks and two days*

Jon walks into our bedroom carrying two newly arrived boxes. "Should I open these?"

I nod before he pulls the new CD player from the cardboard. "This looks great." He inspects it from all sides before leaning over to plug in my newest acquisition.

"I thought some music would be nice." I feel sheepish, looking at the other unopened box, wondering how many more will arrive today.

"What a good idea," he says.

He's been so thoughtful since we last left Dr. Randolph's office, after he asked me to rate our office visit using his proposed scale: a terrifying one to a gleeful ten. I gave it a two. The look on his face said that he'd missed something. But instead of fighting about whose reaction was right, he asked me why I felt that way, and listened carefully when I explained. His eyes widened, then his arms opened.

"How's your back?"

"Still throbbing."

He nods. "Scoot over."

I gladly move to the center of our bed, eager for the company. He nudges me onto my side, and begins rubbing my back.

"It's been forty-eight hours. Does that make you feel any better?" His thumbs knead into the sway of my back.

"A little. If the baby comes, there will be some protection—for the lungs." If only there were other preventive treatments to hedge against all the pitfalls of prematurity, to ensure a healthy life if this baby comes too soon. But the only treatment is time; with each day that I remain pregnant, the baby develops a little more, inches a little further from a mere 40 percent chance of survival and the risk of lifelong disabilities.

"Jon, I've been thinking, about the pregnancy, all the risk. There's such torment, you know?"

"I know."

"Some days I don't know if I can handle it, waiting to see if today's the day I'll lose the baby."

"I know."

"I've decided that I need to make myself a promise—that this is the last time I'll ever be pregnant."

He releases a vexed breath, then moves his hands to my shoulder, clutching the muscle as he stretches my neck to the side. The pull relieves some of the strain that comes from seventeen weeks of bed rest, as does the warmth of him lying beside me.

"It makes sense. It's enough. All of this, it's just enough." He shakes his head as he stretches my neck, gently pushing on the ligaments that attach to the shoulder. "I support you, with whatever you need to do."

His words fall over me like a warm rain. *He supports me.* His old voice starts to speak in my mind, but the words disintegrate before I can even recall them. *My husband supports me.*

I turn toward him and grasp his hand. "That feels better. Thank you."

His lips part with bittersweet contentment. "Why don't I go to the basement and bring up a few boxes of CDs for your player? They shouldn't be too hard to find."

I push the hair from Jon's forehead and stroke his graying temples, think about all the pain and sacrifice we've both endured these past six years, take in the man who lies by me today, doing what he can to give me comfort. I close my eyes and imagine what our life might have been like without the repeated strain of loss and recovery, without such aching knowledge of our mutual limitations. Then I glimpse a future filled with understanding, love, and joy, even if only for the three of us.

JANUARY 12 *Twenty-four weeks and four days*

"I still have the radiating back pain, Dr. Randolph." I stiffen into the cold exam table as he marks another measurement. Jon sits in a chair pulled against the table, holding my hand as he watches.

"Brrr." I shiver. Jon wraps his fleece around my shoulders.

I close my eyes and focus on relaxing as much as possible. Dr. Randolph has said that the cervix is dynamic during pregnancy, that the length can increase or decrease. But the number last week felt like walking on a ledge where all the windows were closing.

"The cervix is fifteen millimeters." Dr. Randolph seems unfazed by the number. "It is consistent with last week."

"And the funneling?" Jon asks.

"The same. The funnel has not retreated from the cerclage." He removes the transvaginal probe and hands it to the technician.

I'd so hoped for relief, to find an open window and step in.

"So there's really no change. We're where we were last week." Jon looks disappointed.

Dr. Randolph gives a quick confirmation before picking up the abdominal ultrasound paddle. The technician splats more jelly on my stomach before he presses the transducer against my skin. The doctor is silent while images click from moving to still on the machine. "The baby does seem sizable for this gestational age. The weight estimates at nearly a pound and a half. That's within the seventieth to eightieth percentile."

Warmth starts to leave my body.

He's estimating the baby's weight.

My eyes flutter as tears trickle out the corners. *He's never estimated the baby's weight before today.*

Birth weight influences survival rates and the long-term outlook for preemies.

He thinks I'm about to have this baby.

~ JANUARY 13 *Twenty-four weeks and five days*

I sit on the exam table in Dr. McConaughey's office. My hands tremble as I wait for him to come in. The door opens, and after he sees me, he sits down.

"I read the notes from your visit with Dr. Randolph yesterday." He looks at me over the top of his squared Italian eyeglasses. "How are you doing?"

"Dr. McConaughey, I'm frightened. It feels like I could have this baby any minute." We talk about my continuing back pain, shortened cervix, and funneling. He then asks me to lie back on the exam table.

He inserts the speculum. I feel the pinch, and the pressure.

"If I do go into labor now, which hospital should I go to?" Dr. McConaughey and Dr. Randolph are at a community hospital, not a major trauma center. Premature babies require special care in a Level III NICU, found only in larger hospitals. Maddie spent nearly two months in one of these specialized units.

"If you do go into labor, you should come here." He explains that for most deliveries before thirty-two weeks, the hospital tries to transport patients to the nearest Level III NICU before giving birth. "If it's not safe to transport, we could deliver here, then move the baby as soon as possible."

I'm overwrought with the possibility of this choice. Will I really have to pick between chancing the longer drive to the better-equipped hospital versus the safety of closeness?

"If the pregnancy is sustained past thirty-two weeks, you may not need a Level III NICU. You and the baby could stay here."

I nod, unable to grasp such an unimaginable possibility. "Dr.

McConaughey, there's one more thing. I never want to be pregnant again. When we do the C-section, I want a tubal ligation." Tiny beads of relief bubble up from my chest.

"You should think about that. You're only thirty-seven. Can you be certain that you will never want more children?"

"I can't be pregnant again. I have to promise myself that I'll never go through this again." I rise up on my elbows. "My husband and I have agreed."

"And are you certain that if things don't end well in this pregnancy—"

"I can never do this again."

He finishes the exam, walks to my file, and studies the pages. "Let's keep talking about this. Tubal ligation is permanent. You need to be absolutely sure."

 JANUARY 14 *Twenty-four weeks and six days*

I don't think I can take much more. My back throbs. My nerves are frayed. I've journaled and read. I've cried and shopped. I've spent hours on the phone with family and friends, the people who help sustain me when reality gets thick and swirling. But nothing conquers the smothering fear that I'm about to lose this baby.

The only thing left is food.

I usually nurture myself with comfort food like mashed potatoes, chocolate cake, or freshly baked bread with butter. Unfortunately we've eaten little else except pizza and takeout and oatmeal since September, the only exception being the few days that visitors came and cooked. If I could have only one hour of freedom from this bed, I would go to my kitchen and cook.

If any of the women in my life were here, they would cook for me. My mother-in-law would make a hearty pot roast. My sister would make a beefy pot of spicy chili. My epicurean friend Kelly would make coq au vin with hot crusty bread for dipping in the rich juices. I would feel nourished, safer.

"Hi, Karen?" I hold the phone gingerly, embarrassed that I'm calling a woman I barely know, a mom from Maddie's school. Karen invited me over before school started. We talked over coffee with frothed milk, freshly diced fruit, and warmed pastries. I imagine her cooking savory meals for her family every night.

She has called to check in a few times since Maddie blabbed about the pregnancy. I've never told any of our neighbors about the bed rest, until now.

"I had no idea," she says. "How long have you been on bed rest?"

I tell her more about this pregnancy, but don't divulge how bad things are right now.

"I'm calling to ask a favor," I finally say. "This feels so awkward. I mean, I barely know you."

"Anything. What can I do?"

"Well, I really need some mashed potatoes. I'm craving them. Not the fancy stuff you get in a restaurant, just the basic stuff, homemade."

"That's all you need?" She starts to laugh. "I could make you dinner—"

"No. Really. I would feel awful to put you through that much trouble. But I just know you're a cook, and I was hoping that the next time you make mashed potatoes you could make some extra. I'll send Jon to pick them up. Whenever it is."

"Absolutely."

I feel relieved, touched that she would do this for me, and warmed by the thought of homemade potatoes. When I get off the phone, I burst into tears.

⟋⟍ JANUARY 15 *Twenty-five weeks*

"You're not going to believe this." Jon and Maddie walk into our bedroom carrying brown bags and plates.

The smell of chicken and pepper and vegetables fills the room. I sit up in bed as Jon starts pulling casserole dishes from the paper bags and stacking them on the toddler table. He pulls the lid from a white Corningware dish and reveals a still-steaming pile of creamy mashed potatoes, speckled with pepper, melted butter cascading from the whipped crests.

"Karen just dropped all this off. Can you believe it?"

My mouth gapes as I survey the table: chunks of chicken in a thick gravy with peas and carrots, a crisp salad with peppers and tomatoes, crusty bread, and of course, mashed potatoes.

There is no conversation during dinner. We all eat like we haven't been fed in a month. After my third helping of potatoes I grab the serving dish and scrape the remnants with a spoon, sliding the end up each corner of the dish.

Maddie's eyes flash as she watches me eat. When all the food is gone, she reaches again into the crinkling bag. "There's one more surprise!"

She beams when she lifts the glass casserole dish to the table, a homemade apple crisp.

"This is so unbelievably nice. I . . . I . . . just can't believe . . . She hardly even knows us." I feel my voice breaking as Jon smiles and serves the warm apples with the crumbled, browned topping into bowls.

I feel comforted, nurtured.

"There's something else in here." Maddie pulls an envelope from the bag. She hands it to Jon.

My husband opens the envelope. His mouth falls open. He hands me the paper.

It's a note from Karen with a schedule of meals for the next two months. This woman I barely know has arranged two months of home-cooked dinners for our family from all the other kindergarten parents.

I feel myself starting to cry, and I feel a little silly until I look toward Jon. His eyes are filling, too.

JANUARY 18 *Twenty-five weeks and three days*

"Maybe we should come in until you get set up. I could take Maddie home later."

I look in the backseat where Maddie looks dazed, having been pulled from her bed at eleven P.M. for another trip to the hospital. The car idles at the ER entrance while I gather my bag. Jon looks tired, and torn.

"I'll call you as soon as I know anything." I clutch my stomach with the stab of another sharp pain. "You can always come back. And I could be here for hours. I'd feel better if Maddie were sleeping."

I watch the car pull away before walking to the ER nurse I now recognize.

~ ~ ~

"My recommendation," Dr. Berkeley says, "is that you go home and get back in bed. Are you comfortable with that?"

Three hours of monitoring have detected no pattern to the

pains that come and go in my stomach. But when the cramping came to accompany the pulsing back pain that's been ongoing for weeks, I came to the ER for monitoring.

I am now twenty-five weeks pregnant, a milestone when survival rates increase to 70 percent. If the baby comes, the odds now favor survival, but the strong threat of long-term disabilities still looms. At this point, the prognosis for my baby improves with every single day that I can sustain this pregnancy. I can't risk ignoring any symptom that may be my only warning to save this child.

"Dr. Berkeley, with the pain, if I had crossed into labor and needed to stop the contractions, if I had needed the medication . . ."

"At this point, you do not need anything to stop contractions. Your symptoms have not crossed that threshold."

"If I do, the next time, how well do the drugs work? Will they definitely stop labor, at least for a few days?" I wait for her response, hoping the reality can quell my helplessness and panic. I want an assurance that the treatments will be ironclad if needed; but because this is medicine, I know I'll likely get something far less.

"The treatments are usually effective at delaying labor. They can often halt the process altogether."

"Dr. Berkeley, I hope you understand." I shake my head as my face dissolves from the constancy of day after dire day. "I had to be sure. I don't want to seem like some sort of nervous Nellie, but I just had to be sure. If I had needed medication to slow things down, if—"

"Darci." She grasps my hand and holds it. "It's okay. Anytime you think something is not right, you should come in. With your history, you need to be absolutely safe."

I nod, appreciating her compassion, indebted that she doesn't see my vigilance as dispensable. I'm reassured that the pain does not yet constitute labor, but I feel crushed by the ever-present fear that at any moment, it will.

JANUARY 22 Twenty-six weeks

Alarms blare on all the monitors attached to Maddie in the NICU.

She's not breathing. Her heart rate is nearly flat.

The nurse screams for help.

Her stats are almost flat.

The doctors run.

The nurse slips a mask over her face and squeezes the blue bag attached.

Please, God, please save my daughter.

The nurse squeezes. Squeezes. Squeezes.

I bolt up from the couch as the *knock knock knock* on the front door rips me from a tortuous afternoon sleep.

"Maddie? Maddie!" I'm panicked, disoriented, somewhere between the reality of my living room sofa and the place I just was in my nightmare, the NICU where Maddie nearly died.

More pounding on the door.

"Maddie!" I scream and run to the door, ripping it open to find a startled parent staring at me with a shocked expression.

"Where's Maddie? Maddie? Is she all right?" My heart pounds and I don't know where my daughter is and I'm seething in fear for her.

"She's in the house. Darci, calm down. I just dropped her off," the parent's mouth gapes.

I nod quickly. *I am in my home. It was a nightmare.* My chest pounds as I fight an explosion of tears that can't come in front of the parent who now stares at me like I'm crazy. I try to speak but I can't.

"Darci, she ran inside when I dropped her off. The door was unlocked, but after she ran in I thought I should make sure someone was here."

It's almost five o'clock. Maddie is just getting dropped off after a play date. She is fine.

"Yes, yes, of course." I spit out the words as I tremble.

"Mom?"

I turn and see Maddie bounding down the stairs, looking bewildered.

"Thank you so much for bringing her home." I drop my head, chest still heaving.

"Should I come in? Are you okay?"

"Fine. Really. Thank you." I close the door and run to Maddie, squeeze her into my arms, touch her hair, her shoulders, her back.

She is fine. Maddie is safe.

Clutch her to my body.

They saved her. It's all over now. She is real. My daughter is here, alive.

〜 JANUARY 25 *Twenty-six weeks and three days*

"Have another one. Come on, enjoy yourself." Ev puts the plate with the second richly frosted cupcake by my bed. Since she and Steve came two days ago I've had two servings of everything. When she comes to take my dishes she automatically brings more if my plate was cleaned. I don't really need the double servings, and I could avoid this if I would simply leave something on my plate. But these days, that's impossible.

My back pain has eased to a lower-grade, intermittent ache. The pain doesn't pulse anymore, but after five weeks of being on the cusp of labor, my nerves are shot. I bite into chocolate frosting, once again turning to food for a moment of relief.

"Are you feeling any better today?" She sits in a chair by my bed, looking content as she watches me eat chocolate powerful enough to soothe two women.

"A little." I wash down the cupcake with gulps of ice-cold milk.

"And the back pain?"

"It's better today. I think it's easing up." I hope this means I can hang on to this baby, at least a few weeks longer for survival rates to further improve. At twenty-six weeks, 75 percent of babies will survive.

Every single day continues to matter in this pregnancy, and I feel blessed that I've hung on this long. I just saw Dr. Randolph a few days ago and my cervix was 19 millimeters, an improvement from last week, but still suggesting a high chance of preterm delivery.

My heart sinks at the thought of having another preemie. I don't know if I'm strong enough to take all the weeks in the NICU again. I remember sitting helplessly by Maddie's incubator when she teetered on the edges of existence, when doctors discussed brain bleeds and sepsis and respiratory distress.

I shudder and look away. Ev notices.

"I . . . well . . . I just keep remembering Maddie, in the NICU."

Ev smooths out her pants and then nods. "Me, too."

I recognize the torment in her eyes, realize that she also saw her share of horrors when Maddie was born. Ev and Steve came to stay with us for weeks, driving me to the hospital to see

Maddie, taking turns sitting with us in the NICU, containing themselves in our presence only to collapse as soon as they passed the hospital exit.

"I don't know if I can get through another stint in the NICU. I barely did it with Maddie—and I was stronger then."

I think about how weakened and anxious I am after months on edge. "How am I going to do this now? I'm so spent. I feel like there's just not much left of me."

She shakes her head. "But you will. I know how strong you are, and if you have to—God forbid, if you have to, you will handle it." Ev looks as though her own resolve has pushed aside her anguish and steeled her to take whatever the next few weeks brings.

I squeeze her hand and find some solace knowing that whatever does happen, she will be with me.

/⟋ JANUARY 29 *Twenty-seven weeks*

"I told Dr. McConaughey I wanted to have a tubal ligation."

I grasp the edges of Dr. Randolph's exam table, again being prodded and measured, waiting for the numbers that will tell me whether I can breathe. I feel a little more stable today—the back pain is gone and I haven't felt cramping for days.

"Is there something in the hospital record about doing the tubal when we do the C-section?" With Maddie I had a classical C-section, meaning the uterus is cut vertically, despite the horizontal incision across my belly. With this specific cut, I face an increased risk of uterine rupture if I deliver vaginally; regardless of when this baby is born, I know that my only choice for delivery is a C-section.

"I have nothing in my records. But that is something you

need to confirm with Dr. McConaughey. As your primary OB, he will be performing the C-section."

My heart jumps at the thought of not having Dr. Randolph do my delivery. I feel a stronger connection with him—and how could I not? I've seen him far more frequently than Dr. McConaughey, and it's Dr. Randolph who faces the worst threats with me.

Jon glances at me from his chair, gripping the arms as though he's about to rise. He shoots Dr. Randolph a confrontational look. I nod him back down, my attentive husband picking up on the exchange that just made me grimace.

I do trust Dr. McConaughey. He's competent and dedicated, and he has shown me real compassion during the visits when my fear fills the room. I try to settle into the knowledge that my baby will be fine in the hands of either capable doctor.

I study Dr. Randolph as he purses his lips and deliberates the images and numbers from the monitor. It dawns on me that I really trust this man. He has listened to every one of my concerns, tried to quell my anxieties, and never once dismissed my fears as ridiculous. After all the specialists and major trauma centers in California, I now lie on an exam table on the opposite coast from where all this started.

Maybe this is simply where I was meant to be.

"The number appears stable." Dr. Randolph looks relieved. "The cervix is twenty millimeters—still well below what we would like—but consistent with last week. And the funnel has receded."

He crosses his arms and slumps against the wall. "As we have seen, the cervix is dynamic. You appear stable at the moment, but this could, of course, change."

Does this mean I can breathe? Does this signal a temporary

reprieve, a sliver of time when I can allow possibility to be tangible?

"I want you back home, and straight back to bed. While you appear stable at the moment, we need to continue with every precaution." He looks at me suspiciously, as though he thinks I may go dancing with my tentative stay.

"Do not change anything that you've been doing."

FEBRUARY

FEBRUARY 1 *Twenty-seven weeks and three days*

I dream of Maddie, my precious little preemie nestled bare inside my shirt, her skin touching my skin. Her tiny chest rises with each breath released through parted pink lips, and I stroke the thin fuzz that covers her head before hair had a chance to develop. I close my eyes to block out all the intrusions of the NICU, making this a private moment between mother and daughter.

Born three weeks ago, she weighs almost four pounds. I look at her tiny body in amazement, gestationally still only thirty-one weeks, her skin so thin she's tinted purple. She sleeps as we rock in the chair next to her incubator, one of the two times each day that I can hold her, feel her warmth, and let her feel mine. I stroke her impossibly tiny forehead, nearly covered by just one of my fingers. It feels cool so I snuggle her closer and button my shirt, weaving her attached wires and leads and cords through the gaps between my buttons. Her face is relaxed. Calm. Limp.

The pulse oxygen monitor blares. Her oxygen has dipped. I notice her pale face.

The heart rate monitor screams as her heart slows.

Both monitors shriek. I try not to panic as her stats drop.

I've seen it before, apnea and bradycardia, a tortuous phase for preemies when their lungs stall and their heart stumbles.

She usually rights herself, her tiny body somehow checking these errors and regaining sync in seconds.

But seconds have passed. She's not righting herself.

I call for the casual and efficient nurse who has seen this a thousand times, always effortlessly rousing Maddie back to normal.

The nurse reaches inside my shirt to shake Maddie while I start to unbutton.

Her stats keep falling. Another alarm sounds, one I've never heard.

The nurse says we need her out of my shirt. She tugs at my blouse.

Her stats keep falling. How long has it been? The nurse screams for a doctor.

Doctors and nurses run. I've never seen them run. I can't get the shirt unbuttoned. My hands tremble the buttons are stuck her cords are tangled in my shirt I can't get them untangled.

Her stats are almost flat.

The doctor grabs my shirt and pulls it over my head while I hold Maddie steady. They rip her from my arms and lay her in the incubator.

The doctor pumps two fingers against her chest and the compressions ripple across her fragile body while the nurse squeezes a blue bag attached to a mask on her face.

How long has it been? My God! She doesn't have enough oxygen. Has it been one minute? Has it been two?

They press and squeeze and press and squeeze and I see her helpless ashen body flinch with each motion.

Please let her be okay. God, please.

Her stats begin to pick up.

I sit motionless while her heart rate climbs and her respiration increases.

Her pulse oxygen climbs toward a normal level.

The doctors and nurses step back from her incubator and whisper.

I clutch the sides of the rocking chair, mouth gaping, chest bare.

The nurse with hands that now shake unbuttons my shirt hanging from Maddie's cords like laundry on a clothesline.

"My daughter is okay," I tell myself over and over.

I breathe and unclutch the sides of the rocker. The nurse gives me my shirt as I stare at Maddie's stats, now normal, objective proof that she rebounded.

But what about the next time?

FEBRUARY 4 *Twenty-seven weeks and six days*

"Look at these ribs!" Jon wears the face of a child at Christmas.

I rest on the couch and watch as Jon and Maddie unpack the latest dinner from our school community, unveiling each of the dishes with flourish before placing them on the coffee table. A bowl of sesame noodles glistens with slivers of scallion and shredded carrots, creamy cole slaw with shades of green and purple cabbage, and a huge tray of beef short ribs, thick with brick-red sauce that barely covers some of the darkened chunks of charred meat.

"I still can't believe this. I feel so spoiled." Families from school have brought us home-cooked meals every night since mid-January. We feel physically and spiritually nourished.

I spy the last rib remaining on the platter, then count the bones already stacked high on my plate. Jon eyes the rib, too.

"Take it," he says.

"No. I've already had enough." I count the bones on his plate and see that I've eaten more than my hundred-and-eighty-pound husband—but I still want the rib.

He grins and puts it on my plate. I sink my teeth in, tearing the meat from the bone.

"The baby must be really hungry tonight. Look at all the food you ate." Maddie stares at my plate, astonished. "How could such a little baby eat so much?"

"The baby gets some of it, Maddie, but Mommy gets more." Jon seems to survey my expanding girth.

I know I'm getting bigger, much more so than with the other pregnancies. But food is one of the very few indulgences I have with this pregnancy, and one of the more effective diversions from the anxiety I still fight every day.

"How big is the baby now?" Maddie bites into her cookie, warm chocolate chips smeared on her lip.

"Maybe about two and a half pounds now." I stretch out my hands about a foot apart to give her a better idea.

The weight is tracking well, around the fiftieth percentile. If the baby comes now, at nearly twenty-eight weeks, survival rates are 90 percent. Still, the threat remains from all the disabilities that frequently plague preemies. My hope is that this child will not only survive, but be able to thrive—a given for most parents, but a real question for the families of preemies.

"I think the baby needs a name." Maddie looks insistent. "We can't just keep saying 'the baby.' "

"I think that's a good idea," Jon says. "But there's one problem. We don't know if it's a boy or a girl."

For the past three years Maddie has asked us to give her a little sister. Despite all her pleas of neutrality, we both know what she's hoping for.

I smile at my daughter, who already embraces her new sibling, getting closer than I can. The idea of a name, a more concrete identity, makes me quiver with vulnerability. I sit with my unease as I listen to their conversation.

"So Maddie, the baby may be a little girl, or it could be a little boy. And you know either one would be fun," Jon adds.

Maddie nods.

"And we will all be happy with our healthy baby—whether it's a girl or a boy. Isn't that right, Maddie?" Jon arches his eyebrows.

"Yes." She nods wildly to enhance the credibility of her answer. "But I want to pick a name for the baby. I think we should call her Jessica."

"But, Maddie, what if it's a boy? We can't call a little boy Jessica." Jon holds back laughter.

"We could change it later. If we have to," she concedes.

"Okay. I think you're right." Jon looks to me and winks. "Jessica it is."

FEBRUARY 6 *Twenty-eight weeks and one day*

"She named the baby Jessica." I laugh with Mary about Maddie's feigned neutrality. "If we have a boy, she may ask to send it back."

"Maddie will love the baby. She's so maternal." Mary sips her coffee before abruptly putting down the cup. "Oh. I don't want to forget . . ." She opens up her bag and pulls out a fistful of DVDs.

"These are some of my favorites. I know you're looking for distractions, so I thought these might help."

"Thank you." Her gesture is so thoughtful. "It looks like we have the same taste in movies." I scan the cases: art films, romantic comedies, and a few dramas.

"I know you said things were 'more stable' on the phone. Are you feeling more confident, or are you still looking for distractions?" She leans back in the leather chair and rests her arm behind her head.

"It goes back and forth. But I am less worried about survival." Despite the ongoing threat of prematurity, after barely escaping milestones that promised only 40 percent survival, my current odds make me feel fortunate.

"The biggest threat now is prematurity. It's unlikely that I'll carry this baby to term." I feel my shoulders tense. "So I'm trying to prepare myself for some time in the NICU."

"After all you've been through . . ." Mary shakes her head. "And you've told me about the NICU . . ."

I nod, remembering the beeps and low hums of medical devices that filled the room where more than thirty babies lay idle under warming lights in incubators; more than thirty babies, but the dominant sounds came from the drone of machines.

"I'm scared for my baby." I pull a pillow tight to my stomach. "But I'm also scared that I just won't be strong enough to deal with it. I'm so drained after the past six months. And the thought of an NICU—all the times when preemies stop breathing, the risk of brain bleeds . . ." I feel myself getting worked up.

I'm sitting with my fear, giving it a voice, waiting for it to leave. But it sits, stubbornly, filling my mind with all the horrors that took my breath six years ago.

Mary leans closer. "I want you to think about another

scenario—and don't think I'm being a Pollyanna here, I know your risk is very real." She pauses. "But try to get a picture in your mind of you and Jon, home with the baby. Never mind whatever happened before you came home with your healthy baby. Just think about that moment, when your baby will be safe. When this will all be over."

I focus and try to arrange the grains of a desired image that feel scattered.

Mary stands up and heads toward the kitchen. "I'm going to make you some tea."

➤ FEBRUARY 10 *Twenty-eight weeks and five days*

"You've gained ten pounds in less than a month." Dr McConaughey's eyes pop as he glances through the vitals collected by his nurse.

"There's definitely some stress eating, Dr. McConaughey. I can't get the thought out of my head that I'm still likely to have another preemie."

We talk about Maddie's stay in the NICU and how perilously she clung to life. Today is the gestational anniversary of her birth; she came at twenty-eight weeks and five days gestation.

"Darci, you're not in the same place as you were with Maddie." He reminds me of the steroid injections completed weeks ago, undoubtedly offering some protection to my baby's lungs. "And look at the care you are getting during this pregnancy. We are monitoring for any signs of preterm labor, and you have been on bed rest for months. Whatever happens, there will not be any surprises this time. We are well prepared for any complications, and we are taking steps to prevent preterm delivery."

This is all true. Maddie had little protection—we didn't know she needed it. I grasp on to the facts that make this pregnancy more protected than all the others, and they do provide hope that this could be different. But the intensity of the devastation already felt so many times refuses to be allayed when such uncertainty still remains.

"I'm certainly not implying that there is no risk. With your indications, you are still at high risk for preterm delivery. But if the baby does come early, we have every reason to believe the prognosis could be favorable."

I'm thankful for his reassurance, but the threat of lifelong disabilities faced by preterm babies shadows his reassurance.

"Dr. McConaughey, we talked about tubal ligation during the last visit. I've done what you asked, I've thought it over. I'm certain that I want to do it."

He steps back and assesses me. "This is a permanent step. You need to be certain that there are no conditions, nothing that might occur"—he waits—"that could make you regret this decision."

I nod, realizing the implications of his counsel. When a baby is premature and doesn't survive, most women crave another child, need another pregnancy to have any chance of healing. I know I would crave another child, too. I also suspect that I would crumble under the mental strain of another pregnancy, especially after yet another loss.

"I know I never want to be pregnant again, Dr. McConaughey. I need the mental buffer. But there's also a practical matter of birth control. I can't take the pill now that I know about the Factor V Leiden."

I took birth control pills for years before I knew about this mutation, never realizing that I was putting myself at risk for thromboembolism—a potentially life-threatening condition when a blood clot forms and then lodges in a vein or an artery. Women with the Factor V Leiden mutation who take oral contraceptives are at greater risk to develop embolisms than noncarriers who take the pill; some researchers say their risk is ten times higher; other researchers believe the risk may be thirty times more. Regardless of just how elevated the risk actually is, the hormones in birth control pills can activate Factor V, creating danger for carriers outside pregnancy, in their day-to-day lives.

"No. You certainly cannot take birth control pills with Factor V." He nods in agreement.

I'm disturbed that doctors will not prescribe birth control pills to known Factor V carriers, but because testing is so rare, obstetricians unwittingly do it every day. Ten million women in the United States carry this mutation, but few know their carrier status. These women ask for and get oral contraceptives every day, despite the potential risk to their health; it's like a "don't ask, don't tell" rule of obstetrics.

Medical journals have spent more than a decade debating whether the general population—both men and women—should be screened for Factor V Leiden because of the increased risk of thromboembolism. The medical community thinks the cost of general screening is unwarranted, but the increased risk faced by unidentified carriers taking oral contraceptives should set this group apart; several hundred carriers on the pill are thought to die from thromboembolism every year.[23] Some of these lives would have been spared if they had known to avoid oral contraceptives. Still, others are wary of increased screening because identified carriers may face difficulty getting medical insurance or life insurance. The debate about increased screening continues to rage, but so far, the voices of millions of unidentified carriers—those who have the most to lose—have been given no chance to weigh in.

"There are other methods of birth control besides the pill."

I sit patiently while Dr. McConaughey reviews my other options and we discuss the success rates of each alternative.

"Dr. McConaughey, I realize there are other options for birth control, but I still want the tubal ligation. I'm having a C-section, you'll be right there, and I want this procedure. How do I make this happen?"

He studies me a moment before asking a nurse to bring a consent form.

"Think it over. If you're absolutely certain you can bring this back at your next visit."

I place the folded paper into a zippered pocket of my purse.

FEBRUARY 12 *Twenty-nine weeks*

"Oh, no! You're going to beat me to the picnic." Maddie pouts when Jon draws a double blue, surpassing her Tigger on the Candy Land board sitting on the coffee table.

"Maddie, there's still a chance that you could win. Daddy may get set back. Look what happened to me?" I lean from the sofa and point to my Eeyore figurine, sent back to the cookie at the first turn after being just steps from victory.

My hopeful rationale does little to dispel her dismay. She picks a card and sits back with crossed arms.

I glance toward Jon with raised brows. He dutifully picks a card and announces that he, too, just got sent back to the cookie. Maddie celebrates while he quickly slips the card to the bottom of the pile. She looks pleased now that her triumph is all but assured.

"Can we take a break for a snack?" she asks.

After five straight family games of Candy Land, we jump on her suggestion.

"I want to make the snack," she announces. "I know you're not going anywhere, Mom." She looks toward Jon. "But you stay here. I want it to be a surprise."

Jon and I giggle as she skips into the kitchen. We hear the sound of her scooting a chair across the floor to reach the cabinets.

"Can you believe her?" Jon says. "When did she get big enough to make her own snack, much less one for us?"

I marvel at our daughter, bright and lively, kind and sensitive, healthy and growing. "Sometimes I'm amazed when I look at her. She's so healthy, so tall—"

"Maybe the tallest kid in her class," Jon adds.

"And I think about where she started." I shake my head. "Three pounds. Twelve weeks early."

Jon eyes me. "You realize that this baby is about the same gestational age as Maddie when she was born."

I visualize the baby inside and imagine another Maddie fixing a snack in six more years.

"I know you're worried, and I understand—what we went through with Maddie was awful." Jon reaches to grab my hand. "But do you see how it can turn out? That even if the baby were born right now, it could be okay?"

"Here it is!" Maddie carries a bowl of popcorn, chocolate M&Ms, and tiny marshmallows. She's crowned her mixture by streaking the top with lines of chocolate syrup. "It's not my recipe. I had it at Denise's birthday party," she confesses.

"It looks wonderful, Maddie. But this is definitely treat food. It counts as dessert for tonight." She agrees as I scoop a handful of her deliriously sweet surprise.

FEBRUARY 13 *Twenty-nine weeks and one day*

Jon sits beside me as I lie on the exam table. Having completed her part of the examination, the technician summons Dr. Randolph with a familiar pound on the wall. As he maneuvers the probe, I feel breathless, like a defendant awaiting a verdict.

"The cervix is about eighteen millimeters." His face is expressionless as he continues to assess different views and adjust different dials.

"So the number is stable from two weeks ago?" I know the answer, but I want to hear it from his lips.

"Yes."

"Is the funneling still gone?" Jon watches the screen from the edge of his chair, no doubt hoping to retain the modicum of relief after our last visit, when the funneling had disappeared.

Dr. Randolph studies the screen and contemplates the question. "The funneling has reappeared, but it is minor." He points to an image that shows the cerclage still intact and in the middle of the cervix. "Funneling is again present here, but the funnel is well above the cerclage." His face looks relaxed, revealing only mild strands of caution.

"I am twenty-nine weeks." I look toward Jon. "We actually made it to twenty-nine weeks." I'm tinged with astonishment as the fact seeps in. "Do you realize that I've never been this pregnant before?"

Maddie was born at twenty-eight weeks and five days gestation. I have now carried this pregnancy, my fifth pregnancy, longer than any before.

Jon grins, no doubt happy to hear me repeating the message he seeded just last night.

"The baby is well grown. Looks to be nearly three pounds. Rather hefty for this point." Dr. Randolph sways as he reviews the numbers.

"That's not as big as Maddie," Jon says. "She was three pounds five ounces when she came at twenty-eight weeks."

"Are you saying that Jessica is a runt?" I jab Jon.

"So you're considering names, are you?" Dr. Randolph's ears perk up. We explain that Maddie has named the baby Jessica, refusing to call her sibling "the baby" any longer.

I glance at Jon. "So do you think we're ready? Are we ready to know whether this really could be a Jessica?"

Jon drops his head with a grateful giggle. We wait to see if the possibility floating between us dissipates.

"Do you want to know the sex?" Dr. Randolph asks.

We check with each other for final confirmation.

"Yes."

"A boy. You're having a baby boy."

Everything just became real. I caress my stomach and close my eyes, wondering whether our baby, our son, can feel the gentle strokes of my fingers that I imagine brushing against the softness of his cheek, stroking down the line of his tiny arm.

A son. I am carrying our son.

FEBRUARY 14 *Twenty-nine weeks and two days*

"Happy Valentine's Day!" Jon carries another homemade dinner into our bedroom, this time clutching a brilliant bouquet of red tulips.

We've gotten each other red tulips every Valentine's Day since our first year in San Francisco. I was rushing from the train at eight P.M. to meet Jon for dinner, an hour later than we'd planned. When I called him in the afternoon, swamped with work, saying I couldn't make our date until later, he was relieved. He'd been contemplating the same phone call for most of the day.

I raced from the train, still without a present, stopping at the florist in the station. Roses were eighty dollars a dozen. Ridiculous, even with my guilt. Then I saw the tulips, red and brilliant, painted inside with the contrast of yellow and black that somehow made them seem feisty.

I hurried to the restaurant where my husband waited. He saw me coming with my bouquet and laughed before unveiling his collection of red tulips, slyly hidden under the white linen tablecloth.

And here he is again, eight years later, still getting me these symbolic flowers. "You took the time to get me tulips. Thank you, sweetheart."

He hands me the flowers, safe in Aquapics, arranged in a gleaming white box. He leans down to kiss me and I crane my neck to make my pearls visible, the glistening strand he bought me for our first Valentine's Day, back in Chicago.

When I dressed this morning, I decided I was tired of baggy sweats and maternity sacks. I put on the low-rise maternity jeans that Jon bought me for Hanukkah this year, and one of my upscale blouses from the box of stylish maternity clothes with price tags still attached. I bought them for the office, six years ago, during my pregnancy with Maddie. Because I gained so little weight with her, I didn't need maternity clothes until twenty-six weeks; because she was born at twenty-eight weeks, just two weeks after my shopping spree, I've never had the chance to wear most of them. I've been waiting to open that box for years.

"You're wearing your pearls." He strokes my face, gazing with the same awe I saw when he latched them around my neck ten years ago.

He stops and grins, then hands me the next box: gourmet chocolates from my favorite candy store. "I got you the three-pound box," he boasts, enabler that he is.

I praise his choice while I pull off the ribbon and find my favorite, a milk-chocolate-covered coconut hive. "The boy loves these. I just know it."

I've used this excuse for every indulgent food eaten in the past twenty-four hours, after discovering I am carrying a son. "Where's Maddie?" I look around, wondering when our daughter will bound through the room.

"I got a sitter for tonight. She's downstairs, so we could have dinner alone."

Jon unpacks the collection of delicacies prepared by a neighbor: chicken braised in a white wine sauce with Mediterranean spices, saffron rice with dices of scallion, and a steaming platter of roasted vegetables that glisten with olive oil. Before he starts to serve, he pops a DVD into the player.

"Entertainment, too?" I beam, warmed to my toes by his thoughtfulness. "What did you get?"

He smiles, but I also see a little gulp. "*Bridget Jones's Diary.*"

My husband hates chick flicks; but for tonight, he has rented this apex of women's entertainment to watch with me. For my husband, who craves adventure flicks and often must do puzzles or scan magazines to stay entertained while watching anything without Bruce Willis, I know this is his ultimate sacrifice.

"Thank you for doing all of this. It's absolutely wonderful." I motion him over for another kiss.

"I'm a little cold. Would you mind grabbing a sweater out of my closet, sweetie?"

He dutifully walks to my closet and opens the door. On the floor are a dozen red tulips arranged in a vase.

He quickly turns, surprised. "How . . ."

"I had them delivered today. I would rather have arranged them myself, but, well—"

"You remembered. In the midst of all of this." He waves his hands and scans the room where I've spent most of the past five months. "You managed to get me tulips."

He carries the vase to his nightstand and places the flowers by his lamp. I take a bite from my heaping plate and rest my head on Jon's shoulder as Bridget shares her first exploit.

➤ FEBRUARY 17 *Twenty-nine weeks and five days*

"So, Maddie. Mommy and Daddy have a very special present for you."

Her eyes light up as she gobbles up dessert, homemade chocolate cake that came with tonight's meal. "What is it?"

Jon walks into the dining room and retrieves the tall package still wrapped in blue and silver Hanukkah paper. Maddie nearly bursts as he sets it in front of her.

"Can I please open it now?"

I nod after her hands have already reached for the gift, and then shreds of paper fly through the air. She holds the box in her hands, Baby Chou Chou visible through the clear plastic window. She squeals in excitement.

Jon helps her loosen the tape and the cords that hold the baby safely in its package. Maddie clutches the doll to her chest.

"Maddie, we thought you needed this doll to practice being a big sister."

Jon reads the package to learn how to activate Chou Chou's special abilities while I market them all to Maddie.

"She's a big responsibility, just like a real baby. She cries when she's hungry or sleepy, and when she does, you'll have to soothe her."

"Oh, I will, I will, Mommy." Maddie picks through the accessories that came with the baby, focusing on the bottle. "I'll need this to feed her."

"And do you see the diaper?" Jon holds up the tiny cotton diaper. It looks like one of the preemie diapers we used in the hospital with Maddie. "You can practice on this baby. Then you'll be ready to change Jessica's diapers."

Maddie looks hesitant. "I can change the pee. But will there be doody, too?"

Even in her elation, she still has her limits. We confirm that there will be both, and that she doesn't have to change any diapers unless she's comfortable. I wink at Jon, and lean in toward Maddie for the next part of our news: She's going to have a baby brother.

She embraces the doll, and I glimpse the two of us caring for our babies, perfecting our mothering skills. My son is already gestationally older than Maddie was. I will have a son. Maddie will have a brother.

"I think I'll name her Julie." She holds out the doll, inspecting her pink jumper and tilting her back and forth to see her plastic arms flop. Jon takes the doll long enough to flip a switch in her back, and Chou Chou begins to giggle.

"I better feed her." Maddie pops the bottle into the doll's

mouth and sucking sounds emerge. "Wow! Jessica will be so happy to meet Julie."

Jon and I both decide to hold the second part of our news.

 FEBRUARY 27 *Thirty-one weeks and one day*

"How severe is the cramping?" Dr. Randolph creates tiny electronic Xs on the screen, then connects them with an electronic dashed line.

"Moderate. On the pain scale, I'd give it maybe a four."

I began feeling uneasy a few days ago, and then last night the cramping came. There is no throbbing back pain yet, but I can feel a slow build brewing in my lower back.

Jon sits on the edge of his chair, scooted up to the exam table. Dr. Randolph's brow begins to stiffen as he takes more measurements. He is not speaking much during this exam. Jon and I trade anxious glances as the gaps of silence grow in length.

"Your cervix has deteriorated again. You are down to fourteen millimeters." Dr. Randolph puts down the probe and picks up my chart. I squeeze Jon's hand while the doctor studies the chart. We are once again below 15 millimeters, when research predicts that 30 to 50 percent of women will deliver preterm.

Dr. Randolph closes the chart and calls our attention to the image on the screen. I recognize the funnel before he points it out.

"How bad is it?" I bite my lip while staring at the stark illustration.

"The funnel descends down to the cerclage." Dr. Randolph pulls his eyes from the monitor as though he has studied it to a point of discomfort.

Now the other harbinger has come, the one that means my membranes are likely to rupture at any time.

The doctor goes back to the base controls of the ultrasound, punches keys, and turns knobs. "The baby does still appear well grown. He is close to three and a half pounds. That is in the fiftieth to sixtieth percentile."

"Wasn't he tracking larger? Around the eightieth percentile?" Jon strains his neck toward the monitor.

Doctor Randolph scans through our chart. He explains that our son's weight has gradually increased every time that he was measured. "The percentiles have hopped around a bit, but in utero weight estimates are only so accurate. The important thing is that we are seeing steady growth."

His words offer some reassurance, but if fetal weight estimates are not very reliable, then how can we be sure my son is growing steadily? The question is critical; when Factor V Leiden becomes active during pregnancy, fetal growth is often impeded, a syndrome known as intrauterine growth retardation. Growth rates are a crucial clue as to whether the mutation has remained dormant or has been activated.

"You already had steroid injections? Am I remembering that correctly?" Dr. Randolph looks apprehensive.

Jon and I both nod.

"At twenty-four weeks," I say.

The doctor releases a subtle sigh. "Well, you are thirty-one weeks along. We have administered preventive treatment to protect the lungs. My advice is that you go back home and get straight to bed. And if there is any progression whatsoever in your pain, you are to return to the hospital immediately."

When Dr. Randolph leaves, I lie still, silent on the exam

table. Jon still clutches my hand, looking beaten, dejected. "I think that was a two," he says, invoking our grading scale.

I rise to my elbows and nod my torn agreement. "But at least we've made it to thirty-one weeks. Maybe that brings all this up to a four."

✒ FEBRUARY 28 *Thirty-one weeks and two days*

"Dr. Randolph said I should come in if the pain got any worse." I arch my back in the hospital bed as the young ER doctor attaches the monitor's elastic band around my belly. It's midmorning. Jon brought me to the hospital when I woke with pain pulsing down my lower back. He waits in a faux-leather recliner with Maddie in his lap. Maddie plays with Julie, her new doll that now sleeps with her and eats with her. She rocks her baby to sleep as they both sit in Jon's arms.

I thought of waiting out the pain at home, seeing if it became worse and more regular before rushing to the hospital. But I know that the drugs to stop labor are more effective before labor has become too strong; if I had waited to see how this develops, it might have impaired the doctor's ability to halt my contractions. I don't know if any treatment will be needed, but if it is, I want to make sure that the treatment has the best chance of working, that my son has each possible day of development.

"Do you have a history of preterm birth?" Dr. Stiller asks.

I review my history with this new physician. Her eyes widen as my story continues.

"So after yesterday, when Dr. Randolph saw that my cervix was down to fourteen millimeters and the funnel was down to the cervix, he told me to come in immediately if the pain became worse. The cramping is worse, and now the back pain is stronger."

The doctor studies my chart, and from her expression she seems to be contemplating exactly what to do with me. She walks to the base of the contraction monitor and adjusts several controls.

"Okay," she starts. "You're probably going to be here for a while. We need to monitor your contractions—"

She stops midsentence. As the pain builds in my abdomen, I know what has her attention. She watches as the machine graphs my cresting pain onto the gridlines of the paper before the contraction diminishes.

"How often do you think you're contracting?" she asks.

"I haven't timed anything. The cramps feel irregular, but my back pain has gotten worse since yesterday."

"The intensity of the abdominal cramping appears mild." She inspects the graph on the machine.

"The cramping isn't horribly painful." I look to the familiar pain rating poster that hangs from the wall. "On your scale, it's maybe a five."

Jon takes Maddie and Julie to the snack shop while Dr. Stiller performs a noninvasive vaginal exam.

"You're going to feel only a little pressure. I'm barely expanding the speculum—just enough to make sure that the membranes have not prolapsed."

I grab the rails of the bed while I listen to her silence.

I am thirty-one weeks pregnant. Our son has a 94 percent chance of survival if he is born now. His odds are likely even greater because of the steroid injections.

I feel the fear. It sits with me, waiting, recalling all the unhappy endings in whispers that flow through my head.

Ninety-four percent chance of survival, I whisper back.

The discomfort subsides as the speculum releases. Dr. Stiller pushes back on the wheeled stool.

"The membranes have not gone beyond the cerclage." She nods.

Jon returns with Maddie as I cover myself with the thin blanket. He glances between me and the doctor before asking what's going on.

"She is contracting, but the membranes still appear intact," she summarizes. "We need to keep her here for observation."

"For how long?" Jon looks shaken.

"That depends on what we see. But I suspect she will be here awhile."

I look toward Maddie, speaking softly to Julie, the only toy we brought because of our rushed exit from the house. I then study my husband, slumping silently in the familiar spouse's chair.

"Why don't you guys go," I say to Jon.

He's exhausted. She'll be bored before long. And while I am apprehensive, I feel like we're doing everything that can possibly be done. Their absence for a few hours will make no difference in our outcome.

"I'll call Mary. You can take Maddie over to play with Grace."

"And then I'll come right back."

"No. Why don't you go to the gym, or get some coffee. Really."

He resists my suggestion.

"Look, you have your cell. If there's any news, I'll call you immediately. Go take a little break." I look at him calmly, rationally. "Besides, if this is really it, I'm going to need you later."

~ ~ ~

"You truly didn't have to come back so soon."

My husband stands in the hospital room, face still red from shooting baskets for two hours. When I called to tell him that I'd had three contractions in the past hour, he returned immediately.

We wait in the quiet room, watching the graph as it trickles from the machine at a pace that feels stationary, like watching to see if a ghastly weed sprouts among blades of flowing grass. I flip through the latest copy of *People*, rereading the same stories as I try not to stare at the scroll. Jon sits with the *New York Times* crossword puzzle, usually a quick exercise for him. He has remained fixated on the same spaces for over an hour.

"How are you doing?" Dr. Stiller walks straight to the contraction graph, stretching out the scroll as she inspects. The lines in her forehead relax as she surveys the grid sheet.

"I haven't felt any contractions in a while. And the back pain feels duller."

I have now been monitored at the hospital for six hours. She says that I am contracting, but the frequency seems to have tapered off.

"We've only picked up one during the last hour," she confirms.

I nod and take a drink of water. From the moment I got here, the nurses have come every half hour to make sure that my water pitcher was full and that I was drinking. Whenever preterm labor is suspected, one of the first courses of action is hydration. I think I've drunk more water than a horse after a race.

"Do you think she's in labor?" Jon stands by my bed.

The doctor doesn't believe I am in active labor. "But there's clearly some agitation going on." She explains that I may be fine with hydration and rest, or that my contractions may return.

"I feel like I'm in pregnancy purgatory, Dr. Stiller." I look around the familiar room I've now seen four times in this pregnancy, the observation room that separates discharge from admission. My symptoms have eased since this morning, but have not disappeared. I continue to straddle the line between sustaining my pregnancy and meeting our son, before we're certain he'll be safe.

She smiles and nods. "So what would you like to do?"

Dr. Stiller says that I can either go home and return if the pain increases, or she could admit me for overnight observation.

Jon and I discuss the options.

Ninety-four percent survival rate at thirty-one weeks. My son has had steroid injections to protect his lungs.

"We're only minutes away. And since we're just resting and waiting for right now, I think I'd rather go. Is that okay with you?" I check in with Jon.

"I think we'd like to go home," he says to the doctor. "I'll put her right to bed, and if there's any change, we will be back."

MARCH

"I tried to think this through, but I want to make sure you have everything. Is anything missing?" Mary surveys the family room in her home with discernment. The chenille sofa is piled with pillows and blankets, and our favorite morning treats wait on a bronze tray atop the trunk used as a coffee table.

When we talked last night, I mentioned how tired I'd grown of my own four walls after nearly six months of home confinement. It's starting to feel more like house arrest at this point, but without the certainty that I'll be fully pardoned when my sentence ends; my term may be extended to include anguish with no end date. Because the cramping and back pain has eased, Mary suggested that we do our weekly visit at her house. I felt uneasy, like I'd be taking some wild chance. Then the fear subsided, and I felt butterflies.

I snuggle into her couch with a mixture of gratitude and apprehension as I pull the blanket over my legs. "This was such a great idea. And I know this must sound lame"—I shake my head and speak just above a whisper—"but it feels almost decadent, like a road trip."

There are few things that feed my well-being more than girls' getaways. I try to do spa days with my closest girlfriends, weekends in the city, and once I traveled with three of my dearest friends to a Napa bed-and-breakfast for decadent days of food and wine and gab. This is the first time that lying on a friend's couch counted as an excursion with one of the girls.

"Thank you so much for inviting me over and picking me up. You rescued me from my own four walls."

"Now that you're here, are you still comfortable going out? No second thoughts?" She stands stiff and ready, as though she may swoop me back into the car if I have any misgivings.

It was less than five minutes in the car—less time than it takes to get to the doctor's office. And Mary even had the passenger's seat fully reclined for me. I take a deep breath and sink deeper into the down pillows that bulge under my head. "Mary, I'm glad I'm here. And I can't imagine that lying on my own couch gives me any more protection than yours—but this certainly is nicer."

The twill in the kilim rug anchors red leather chairs to an inviting cocoa sofa, butter-colored walls, and harlequin silk curtains. The space is completed with family candids in demure frames, and baskets of toys and games neatly line one wall. The whole room invites me to come right in and rest—an action that feels awkward even between close friends. And Mary recreated this warm room from a picture she ripped from a magazine. I absolutely love it.

"That's how I put together all my rooms." She says this like there's no other way, as if anyone could do this.

I nod as though her suggestion could be useful to me, despite my complete lack of instinct for decorating. Left on my own, I could never put together such a cohesive room, not with a whole stack of magazines, not even with a blueprint.

"I'm happy to see you more relaxed." Mary grabs her coffee and slouches into one of the red chairs.

"I am feeling more at ease. There's still risk, but at this point, it feels a little less scary." At thirty-two weeks, 95 percent of babies survive, and although the threat of long-term disabilities is still present, it's now greatly reduced. "I feel like I can breathe now." I pinch a piece of blueberry scone. "And I even get a road trip." I grin appreciatively.

"So you can finally let yourself believe a little." She looks relieved, contented.

I nod, cautiously.

➤ MARCH 4 *Thirty-two weeks*

"You're not really all that interesting to me anymore." Dr. Randolph says this matter-of-factly, as if I mean nothing to him.

I've never been so happy to hear these words from a man in my entire life. His quip makes me grin. If Dr. Randolph is making jokes, then I really must be out of danger.

"You've made it to thirty-two weeks. Your cervix is twenty millimeters. And there is currently no funneling."

Dr. Randolph crosses his arms and leans casually against the wall. "You can prop yourself up a bit. You don't have to lie flat all the time anymore."

"You mean I'm off bed rest?" My mouth gapes.

"No. Absolutely not. You're still on bed rest." His face is painted with apprehension. He begins a mild rant. "Now this is where women get themselves into trouble. You think that just because you've made it to thirty-two weeks that you're free and clear. You're not." He puts his hands on his hips and begins lecturing into the air.

"We don't want the baby to come now. The lungs still may not be fully developed." He looks toward me. "And your son could still have other consequences of prematurity at this stage."

I temper my enthusiasm. "So what exactly can I do differently?"

He starts with all the things I still can't do: no housework, no laundry, and his consistent exhortation since September, no sex. "And I don't want you up and running about town, either." He looks toward me with mild vexation.

I meet his annoyance with a nod of agreement, but the voice in my head whispers statistics that make me sit up on the table, where I can speak with him face-to-face.

Thirty-two weeks. Ninety-five percent chance of survival. No signs of imminent labor.

"You can get up and get dressed in the morning. Take a long shower. Lie about on the sofa. You know, like a sick person instead of a woman on strict bed rest."

Good heavens. I've been promoted to "sick person." "So I can be up for brief intervals?"

I sense his reluctance. "Yes. Brief."

My son is protected. I believe that my son is safe.

"Can I go out to lunch?"

The words slip from my mouth as the possibilities race through my head. I start mentally dressing myself in some of those fancy maternity clothes that have languished in their box. I will go—

"You may *not* go out to lunch." Dr. Randolph studies me with alarm and doubt, perhaps regretting the release of optimism that now lingers in the room. "You cannot sit up completely. You can prop yourself up at an angle. For brief intervals." Dr. Randolph seems on the edge of offense.

I remember the couch at my local Starbucks. The plush purple couch is stuffed with full pillows, and it looks out onto the street where people walk and drive and go about the business of their lives. "Okay, Dr. Randolph, I hear you. I will absolutely not go to lunch."

He looks relieved.

"But how about coffee?"

Now he's frazzled.

"Just for fifteen minutes. Just one cup of coffee. You said I could be up for a few minutes. And there's a couch at my Starbucks where I could lie back; I wouldn't be sitting straight up."

He drops his arms to his sides, but still stares with apprehension.

"Dr. Randolph, it has been nearly six months since I've been out in public for anything other than medical appointments. I just want to see people who aren't wearing lab coats and scrubs, and walk into a room that doesn't smell like disinfectant. Just fifteen minutes. Please." I haven't pleaded with anyone for permission since I was a teenager. It's like I've been demoted, stripped of my womanhood, left to deliver an agonizing plea for one damn cup of coffee.

A grin creases his lips. Dr. Randolph now seems more at ease. Whether it was the persuasiveness of my argument or the desperation in my voice, I see his acquiescence before I hear the magic words.

"Okay. You can go."

Oh, yes! I am in near disbelief. This morning I was a helpless woman, but later today, I become a woman who coffees—for fifteen luxurious minutes.

"But no more than fifteen minutes," he admonishes.

"Of course not. I'll go home and rest for a few hours. I won't go until later."

"And you should be reclining, not sitting straight up."

"Uh-huh. I'll lie back on the couch." The Starbucks couch, the one where I can see people.

Dr. Randolph delivers one last preventive glower before leaving the room. I immediately grab my cell to call Jon with the good news.

"You're never going to believe what just happened!"

He takes a second to respond. "Is it bad?"

"No—I get to go out."

I tell him about my appointment and my approved fifteen-minute excursion for coffee. When I'm done, he is silent.

"Darci, are you sure this is okay?"

We review all the stats from today's appointment: stable cervical length, no more funneling, no pain. There's a long pause before I hear his acquiescent sigh.

~ ~ ~

"You wait right here until I come get you." Jon leaps from the car and bounds inside as I watch from the reclined passenger seat of our car.

It has been four hours since Dr. Randolph finally agreed to my fifteen minutes of freedom, of public participation; I had to work nearly as hard to persuade my husband. We are parked in front of Starbucks, in the space closest to the door. I take it as a good sign that the nearest space was open and waiting for us. Jon returns in moments.

"Check your watch. What time is it?"

I glance down. "It's a little after two."

"That's not good enough." Jon grabs my wrist, no doubt regretting his tendency not to wear a watch. "It is exactly 2:08. We are leaving at exactly 2:23. Okay?"

"Absolutely." I nod earnestly.

He holds my arm and helps me out of the car, leading me straight to the empty sofa. As he wedges pillows down my back to make an angle, a young woman with an orange streak through her black hair watches suspiciously from a café table. Another woman sips coffee while turning newspaper pages that crinkle under her fingers, while a middle-aged man keyboards with an intensity that blocks the world around him. My skin tingles as I relish the sight of these mundane activities like pristine snow just after a fierce storm.

Jon grabs a chair and props up my feet as I recline on the couch where the world dances around me. He asks what I want before walking toward the line, returning promptly with a decaf grande, two raw sugars, whole milk and cinnamon, stirred until the sugar is fully dissolved.

"Thank you so much, sweetheart. This is wonderful."

He got nothing for himself. He sits on his hands while he watches me sip. "What time is it?"

I carefully study my watch. "It's only 2:14."

"Are you sure?" He reaches for my wrist.

"Jon, I'm sorry if this makes you nervous. I really don't want to make you uncomfortable. But I've been lying on my back, isolated from anything normal and public for twenty-six weeks.

I desperately need a little taste of ordinary life, even for just a few minutes."

"I know. I know."

"We're at thirty-two weeks. And Dr. Randolph said there are no signs of imminent labor. I would not be doing this if it didn't feel absolutely safe." I give his hand a squeeze.

He relaxes a little, and then sits back. I sip the coffee—decadent, luxurious, as I glance across the faces that go about their daily lives. The woman with the orange hair still sits, tossing fleeting glimpses my way.

"Why is she looking at us?" I lean over and whisper to Jon. Do I look peculiar, an oversized pregnant woman rushing into a Starbucks to lie on the couch like a baby walrus?

"I . . . I . . . She had to move."

"What?"

"She was on the couch when I came in. I told her she had to move."

"You evicted her from the sofa?"

He gives me a wry smile, his inner New Yorker still on call as needed.

I lean in closer and kiss his cheek. "Thank you."

Jon takes a deep breath.

I lean into the couch and nestle a pillow under my neck. Light jazz floats through the air as people fly by outside with briefcases and strollers and backpacks, flow in and out of the store. The sky is brilliant, a spring blue as clear as tropical water. And the sunlight, blazing and luminous, makes even the sidewalks glow in a glistening silver.

I take another drink of coffee. Jon still rests on the sofa, but he nervously taps his shoe. I glance at my watch. "It's 2:20. We should go."

"You have three more minutes." He sits up, seeming both relieved and torn. "We don't have to go yet."

"It's okay. We can go. But there is one quick thing." I pull our camera from my purse. "Can you take a quick shot? I may need to remember this over these next few weeks." Jon laughs while I stand in front of the store display, holding my coffee like a trophy after an arduous race. "Thank you. This was absolutely the best cup of coffee I've ever had." Jon snuggles me into his shoulder as we walk to the car.

MARCH 10 *Thirty-two weeks and six days*

I stand in front of the medicine cabinet and remove the prepackaged heparin injection from the box. While the daily shots are routine at this point, I still dread each time the needle pierces my skin.

Even with the injections, our son still faces risk from Factor V Leiden. Studies have shown that most treated women who carry this mutation have a healthy live birth. *Most.* When loss does occur, it's often in the second or third trimester; one study found that carriers are nearly eight times as likely as noncarriers to suffer multiple losses in these later trimesters.[24] The same study said that mutated women are also three times as likely as noncarriers to endure a single late loss.

I often lament the risk this mutation poses to my son, but I also face risk from Factor V Leiden, even outside pregnancy. Carriers—whether male or female—have a higher chance than noncarriers of developing blood clots than can lead to deep-vein thrombosis or pulmonary embolism. When detected, these clots are usually treatable, avoiding the unnecessary deaths that can result when clots remain unchecked. One of the keys to detection and treatment is educating patients on the symptoms of blood clots and identifying the presence of personal risk factors—including mutations such as Factor V Leiden—so that people at risk know to recognize the signs and seek treatment before it's too late.

David Bloom, the NBC correspondent who died of pulmonary embolism while covering the invasion of Iraq, carried the Factor V Leiden mutation. He was unaware of his carrier status and was said to disregard the pain deep in his leg that signaled his thrombosis, the technical name for blood clots.

My hips are still purple and blue from the months of injections, but I've become somewhat immune to the sting of the medication seeping through my flesh. In seconds the injection is over: an act so brief it takes only a few blinks of the eye, but of such paramount importance that it could make the difference between life and death for my son, and possibly for me.

Because of the link between Factor V Leiden and thrombosis—an event with potentially critical consequences—several medical associations recommend testing for this mutation if women suffer suspicious pregnancy loss. The American College of Chest Physicians, the medical association that sets care standards for pulmonologists, recommends testing for Factor V Leiden after recurrent miscarriage, or even after just one late loss.[25] And the American College of Medical Genetics recommends Factor V Leiden screening for women who suffer recurrent pregnancy loss.[26] But after pregnancy loss, women are not usually treated by pulmonologists or geneticists; they are treated by obstetricians.

The American College of Obstetricians and Gynecologists (ACOG), the group that sets the medical standards in obstetric care, explicitly states that testing for Factor V Leiden is not required after multiple miscarriages before fifteen weeks gestation.

They do say that testing should be considered for losses beyond fifteen weeks, but only when no other explanation can be found.[27] This means that if *any other cause* is suspected, testing for Factor V Leiden need not be completed.

But what happens to women like me who could only identify several possible suspects for their loss, but could never pinpoint a definite, single cause? Under ACOG guidelines, I would be treated only for cervical incompetence, betting my son's life that no other culprit lurked to steal him away. And what would happen to the son I now carry if the obstetric community's gamble was wrong?

MARCH 17 *Thirty-three weeks and six days*

"Mommy!" Maddie sobs while clutching her doll Julie, bursting through the front door with our babysitter, just back from the pediatrician's office. She runs to me where I rest on the couch, throwing her arms around my neck.

"She hasn't stopped crying since the doctor swabbed her throat." Rebecca, the newest babysitter, looks at Maddie with a mixture of sympathy and frustration. "He said she has strep throat."

"It hurt, Mommy. He poked me with a stick and it hurt."

"I'm sorry, sweetheart." I hold her close, rocking her back and forth, but careful to keep her face turned away from my mouth. I stroke her hair and talk in my most soothing voice. She quiets and rests on my shoulder.

"Maddie, you should let your mommy rest here. Why don't we go to your bed, and I could tuck you in with Julie?" Rebecca strokes Maddie's back, trying to lure the contagious child away. Maddie doesn't budge.

When Maddie is sick, she only wants Mommy. I usually cuddle with her, play games, tell stories, anything to make her feel better until she's well. As a toddler she had a severe case of rotavirus and cried if I left her side. We slept together on the guest futon for three straight nights, her sleeping on my chest, until she was better.

I want to stay by her all day, lay cool cloths across her feverish forehead, feed her medicated freezer pops to ease her throat, and lull her into long naps by stroking her face and singing her soft songs. But I now have another baby to protect, the son that could become distressed from the fever and dehydration that may come if I contract Maddie's illness.

"She can stay here for now." I hold her closer and consider my dilemma.

"I'll go get her prescription filled," the babysitter says. "Is there anything else I should get while I'm out?"

"Ask the pharmacist if they have surgical masks, something I could wear over my face so I don't catch her strep."

The sitter examines me like I'm a little crazy before she leaves for the drugstore.

"Okay, Miss Maddie. You get on that end of the couch and I'll stay on this end until Rebecca gets back." I turn on her favorite video. "But when she's back, we can snuggle up and read together. Is that okay?"

She crawls to the opposite end of the sofa and lays Julie on her shoulder, covering up with her favorite blanket. She then starts to speak softly to Julie. "It's all right, baby girl. I'm going to take good care of you, and you'll feel better." She pulls the blanket high over both of their shoulders.

~ ~ ~

"How high is her fever?" Jon asks.

"It's down, about 101 when I last checked."

Jon and I talk on the phone. He called to check on her during a break between his meetings, and I've filled him in on Maddie's bug, and how we've arranged to safely snuggle during her sick day. He gets quiet.

"Are you worried about me being so close to her? I am wearing the mask, so it should be okay."

"No. That's not it."

"I can tell that something's bothering you. What is it?"

"Well, it's just that . . . I arranged a surprise for you. For today."

Jon has heard me lament my appearance for weeks. I'm starting to look in the mirror and notice my scraggly graying hair that hasn't been cut since August, and my toes that haven't been polished since the summer. The latter is especially important to me. My toes are always red, almost a personal trademark. Once when Maddie was three, she walked into my bedroom just after I had taken off the polish. She began pointing and screaming in alarm; she had never seen my toes when they weren't red.

"I thought you might like a manicure and a pedicure. So I found someone to come to the house. Today."

I bite my lip as I imagine the manicurist at my door, her face filling with alarm when she sees the sick child and masked pregnant woman. "That is so nice of you. Jon, that was so thoughtful." I savor the kindness of his gesture, and my cheeks start to flush.

"I know how Maddie is when she's sick. Is she going to let you loose for an hour?"

I glance down at Maddie, snuggled into my shoulder, waiting patiently for me to pick up the Junie B. Jones story where we left off.

"Thank you so much, sweetheart. I can't tell you how much it means to me that you did this." I'm overwhelmed with craving for my husband right now, to throw my arms around his neck and hold him so tightly that it's hard to breathe. "If it doesn't work today, I can reschedule it for later. Either way, you made my day."

~ MARCH 22 *Thirty-four weeks and four days*

"How was that coffee?" Dr. Randolph grins as he studies the ultrasound screen, assessing the images and measurements on the screen for the last time. At thirty-four weeks, I no longer need the specialized care of a perinatologist; this will be my last visit with him.

"The coffee was amazing. I only stayed for fifteen minutes, Dr. Randolph, just like I promised—but it was spectacular."

He looks satisfied.

I've been so tempted to go out, take another fifteen minutes for a coffee, or maybe just walk into a bookstore and smell the books. But I've been a good patient, and a protective mother to the son I nurture from within.

"The cervix is at seventeen millimeters," he says with no intonation. This would have been scary ten weeks ago—and in fact, it was. But this far along gestationally, the figure has been reduced to a mere number, not an ominous warning.

We actually make small talk as he adjusts the ultrasound knobs to do one last check on my son's heart rate. The reassuring numbers pulse across the screen. *132. 128. 130.*

We study the screen, almost bored, like patiently sitting through the previews before the movie begins.

74. 56. 42.

"What was that?" I rise to my elbows.

Dr. Randolph's face cinches and his eyes widen.

58. 58. 72.

Our chatter ceases.

102. 121. 126.

I hear Dr. Randolph exhale, but the breath is shallow, still burdened.

"What just happened to my son's heart rate?"

"There was a brief heart rate deceleration." He stresses that the deceleration was fleeting, that my son's heart rate has returned to normal. "Look at the numbers." He points to the screen, which now offers a steady stream of expected observations.

"But why did that happen?"

"It's likely nothing," he begins, "but it can signal fetal distress. Just to be on the safe side, I would like you to go to Labor and Delivery for a nonstress test."

~ ~ ~

I rest in the Labor and Delivery recliner with the elastic band strapped once again around my waist. The machine records every heartbeat. When my son moves, his heart rate accelerates temporarily.

"We call this a reactive test, when the baby responds after movement," the nurse with the kind eyes and soft hands explains.

I stare at the monitor for more than an hour, watching every number. While I wait, the machine picks up two contractions.

"The intensity was mild. It could just be Braxton-Hicks," the nurse says, referring to the common pains thought to be nature's way of practicing for actual labor. I repeat her reassurances in my head, reminding myself that at thirty-four weeks, there's limited risk from preterm delivery. However, the threat from Factor V Leiden will remain until the moment this baby emerges from the mixed safety of my womb.

My son has no more heart rate decelerations while we watch.

"If there were a problem, if I'd developed a clot that was threatening my baby, there should have been more decelerations—is that right?"

She pauses for a moment. "That sounds logical, but I've never gotten that question before."

I sit rigidly in the chair, still staring at the numbers as though they could reveal my future in complete detail.

"Would you like me to call Dr. Randolph and ask him the question?"

My tension starts to ease. "Yes. Please."

I am thirty-four weeks. My baby is fine.

132. 132. 127.

I am getting treatment. My son has protection against Factor V Leiden.

129. 133. 131.

I am going to give birth to a healthy son.

"I have Dr. Randolph on hold." The nurse returns from the nurses' station. "He said that you're right, that if there was a cause of fetal distress, we would have likely seen more decelerations."

I take a deep breath.

I will be the mother of a healthy baby boy.

"He wants to know if you would like to speak with him, or go back up to his office." She waits patiently for my response.

My son is safe. I believe my son is safe.

"No. Tell him thank you, but I think I'm good."

"Would you like to stay a little longer, watch the numbers a few more minutes?"

I look around the quiet room where empty chairs wait for the next concerned woman to come. "No. I'm ready to go home."

We begin to unlatch the band and disconnect the monitoring cords when an epiphany hits me. I look up at the nurse, and I'm suddenly on the verge of tears.

"Is something wrong?" She steps back.

"I'm thirty-four weeks pregnant. I made it to thirty-four weeks." My jaw drops as the nurse looks on in confusion. At thirty-four weeks, my son shouldn't need a Level III NICU; we've all likely avoided the horror of the NICU. "I can actually deliver here, in a normal hospital."

I tell the nurse about my only living daughter's stay in the NICU, and how I've never been this pregnant, having never made it beyond twenty-eight weeks with any of my other five children. "I never thought this was a real possibility. I'm not even sure what a normal maternity ward is like." I shake my head. "I've visited friends after they've had their babies, but . . . I can only remember the NICU, with Maddie . . ." My head fills with the blare of past alarms when her breath paused and her heart rate slowed, the clamor when the doctors and nurses ran, the fear that made me shake—but all the terror suddenly feels more distant.

Her eyes soften and she pats my hand. "Would you like a tour while you're here?"

I have to pause before standing to follow her through the halls. My steps feel surreal, like I'm walking with someone else's legs, seeing through someone else's eyes. "Can I go see the observation room?"

"If that's what you want to see." She looks surprised.

I follow her down a long hallway toward a room at the end

of the corridor with big glass windows. I walk faster. I want to see the babies—all the glorious babies.

When we get there, the room is empty.

Two nurses scribe charts at a desk and drink soda while they chat about their weekend plans. Three unused Plexiglas cribs are pushed against a wide window where sunlight streams in. The nurses pause a moment when we enter, leaving the room silent without their chatter.

"But the babies? Where are all the babies?" My eyes dart across the barren room.

"They're with their mothers."

My face ripples with bewilderment.

"The babies stay in the mothers' rooms. The mothers are taking care of their babies." She says the second sentence slower than the first.

"But what about the monitors? The alarms? How will you know when one of the alarms goes off?"

She looks confused.

"There are no alarms," she says after a long pause.

The chatting nurses now pretend to work as they listen to our conversation. The words of my guide start to sink in.

There are no monitors.

There are no alarms.

I begin to nod slowly. The nurses resume their work. My docent watches me.

I thank the nurse for the tour and walk myself out. As I walk through the maternity ward hallway, I peek into quiet rooms where mothers stare lovingly into the faces of newborns who freely nurse without the tatters of cords or leads. The mothers hold these precious children closely, and speak in tender voices that can only caress tiny newborn ears. Their carefree whispers float out into the hall and glide over my face like the first out-door breeze after a long bout of infirmed seclusion.

↗ MARCH 23 *Thirty-four weeks and five days*

"Have you had any symptoms since yesterday?" Dr. Mc-Conaughey presses the audio fetal heartbeat monitor that's the size of a pen against my stomach.

I report no cramping, no back pain, no indication of any continuing problem. "And the baby has been moving regularly." After I got home yesterday, I did record the time whenever I felt him move. The activity was frequent, but didn't feel frantic or distressed. By around eight o'clock, I put the pencil down.

"Last night he kept pushing his little feet underneath my rib cage, like he was trying to pry his way out." I never realized how uncomfortable the third trimester can get as the tiny legs grow stronger and more active, kicking and pushing with enough force to sometimes make me grab my belly or my ribs. I relish every twinge and ache.

"I reviewed the nonstress test from yesterday. It appeared normal." He nods. "You've had no symptoms since yesterday, and the baby has been active, so I don't think you have anything to worry about." Dr. McConaughey reminds me of the many tests that suggest my son has no congenital abnormalities, a risk even further diminished by carrying him for nearly thirty-five weeks. "Since you're no longer under Dr. Randolph's care, I need to see you every week. If you have any problem, any symptom whatsoever, you are to call me right away."

I nod and press down the paper gown that doesn't spring back when I move. "Dr. McConaughey, I'm feeling like my baby will be okay, but I do still have some anxiety about the Factor V

Leiden." We talk about the risk that still remains because of this mutation. I think about the research studies in which most treated women gave birth to a healthy son or daughter. Dr. Mc-Conaughey reminds me of my son's steadily increasing weight, a finding that suggests the mutation has not become active. Despite the reassurances, and despite my treatment, I remain painfully aware that clots could develop at any time, and even at this late stage of pregnancy, no one can guarantee my baby's safety.

"We need to keep you on anticlotting medication until six weeks after delivery. You're at increased risk for thromboembolism until then."

"That sounds fine." I sit up on the exam table, waiting for my signal that the appointment is over. He continues to survey my file. Then he looks up with warm green eyes that almost seem playful.

"So at this point, you can start getting up."

What? Did I just hear him correctly? "You mean I'm off bed rest?"

"Yes. But I still want your activity restricted. If you got back to a normal routine you would likely have the baby right away. But you can be up for a few hours each day."

"Can I do our grocery shopping?"

"Yes. But no lifting." He raises his eyebrows. "Someone needs to carry your bags."

"Can I make dinner?"

"If you keep it simple. Don't spend hours standing in the kitchen."

I can shop. I can cook. The domestic chores that once felt onerous and monotonous now feel like an expectant luxury.

"You still need to mostly rest during the day. But you can go out a little—no more than two hours each day."

I stiffen my arms against the table, ready to leap off and dress the moment he leaves. After 192 days on bed rest, most of them spent lying completely flat, watching helplessly as others cared for me and my family, I can now get up. Coolness trickles through me as if someone just opened a window. "When can I start?"

"Today."

~ ~ ~

I arrive early, far enough in advance to get a close parking space along the street that's crowded with cars for the three o'clock dismissal. As I lumber toward the door where kindergartners are released, parents look first with surprise, then elation. The many parents who fed our family for months huddle around me, listening to my update, showering me with encouragement. I swell from their enthusiasm and support.

Within minutes, the door is opened and five- and six-year-olds strapped with backpacks pile out in a single-file line that turns to chaos as soon as they see their parents, splitting like a bunch of atoms crossing in random directions. In the middle of the pack walks a girl with two red ponytails and freckles and a look of indifference as she takes her time among the children who burst past her.

And then she sees me.

Her mouth drops. She screams and throws down her backpack, runs at full speed straight for me. Our excitement floats and joins in the middle, making an invisible tunnel that parts the children and parents that separate us. I lower myself to my knees just before she's there to throw her arms tightly around my neck. I hold her and squeeze her and rock back and forth, my beloved daughter securely in my arms.

"Let's go home," I whisper into her ear. Two parents rush over to help me up from the knee squat that seemed like a good idea—and it was, fifty pounds ago.

"Are you allowed to do this?" Maddie looks through her joy with disbelief.

"Yes. I am now allowed to do this. And I'm coming back tomorrow to do it again." She tightly clasps my hand, all the way to the car.

MARCH 25 *Thirty-five weeks*

The dim lighting in the windowless room makes it hard to see the lunch menu in the Italian restaurant just minutes from our house. I noticed this place when we moved here, and thought it could be a favorite lunch spot on the days when Jon could spare the time. We've ordered takeout many times, but this is the first time I've seen the faux Italian décor of antiqued golden walls with Beaux Arts posters in sturdy black frames.

I hold the menu far out in front of my face, too vain to put on reading glasses on my first lunch date with Jon since September. I dressed up in a red silk blouse with a dark maternity skirt and black suede boots, the only nonmaternity item I could possibly force onto my still expanding body. My hair is in a ponytail, the sole solution for a layered cut that hasn't been trimmed since August. And I dug through my cosmetics to find the red lipstick that usually gets worn twice a year.

Jon giggles at me across the booth, holding my fingers. "So this is what it's like to take your wife out to lunch."

We both nod in agreement and disbelief.

The waitress comes to take our order, friendly, but casual—like we're just one of the hundreds of people she'll see today. Little does she know that other than my family, she is the only other person I'll see, having chosen lunch with my husband for today's lone outing.

Jon leans in as she leaves. "Are you ready to talk about names?"

I grin. We told Maddie just last night that she's having a baby brother. We were braced against the sofa, armed to sell her on the idea of a boy, knowing that she has envisioned a baby sister for several years. When she heard our news, she leaped with joy. We now have consensus that Jessica is off the list. "I'm not sure how to do this, but if we don't think of some possibilities fast, Maddie will beat us to it."

We haven't had a lot of practice with picking names. When Maddie came so early, we hadn't even thought about it. We hemmed and hawed while the hospital clerk who typed birth certificates stopped by our room every day, the room where Jon slept every night until I could go home. It wasn't until four days after her birth, when we'd written and scratched out names on the top of a white cardboard bakery box, that we could finally respond to his persistent question.

"Let's just throw out some possibilities. What do you say about Adam?" Jon looks charged for the discussion.

"No." I say this instinctively, without pausing for the politically correct level of evaluation. "Sorry, sweetie, but it doesn't feel right."

He nods. "Jacob?"

I cinch my nose, but wait before speaking. "It's a great name, but I had this awful boyfriend named Jacob. I have a bad association."

Our salads come as we continue to throw out possibilities that the other dislikes out of pure preference or some obscure linkage to people we barely knew in high school or college. By the end of the meal we have two possibilities: Our son will be a Josh, or a Sam.

➤ MARCH 29 *Thirty-five weeks and four days*

"Today's exam looks good." Dr. McConaughey scans my chart one last time before recapping his latest findings. He then grills me about how much activity I'm getting.

"I am being a good patient, Dr. McConaughey. I'm still resting most of the time, and I'm only up for a few hours each day. Promise."

He grins while scribbling something in my file. "Just to be absolutely safe, I want you to have another nonstress test at Labor and Delivery this week."

"But I'm not having any symptoms right now."

"I realize that. But with the volatility of your pregnancy, let's be on the safe side." He gives a paternal nod. "And one more thing. Are you busy on April thirteenth?"

I laugh at his question. "Nothing that can't be moved, I'm sure. What did you have in mind?"

"I had something open up on my surgical schedule, and I know you're still anxious about the Factor V Leiden. Would you like to move up your C-section to the thirteenth?"

I can hardly believe his words. I've felt less fearful the past week, now able to distract my worries with brief daily jaunts. But I still think about the lingering risk to my son, the threat that remains each day until he's delivered. My C-section is scheduled for April 16, when my son will be just past thirty-eight weeks.

Dr. McConaughey says he would prefer that I wait the extra few days, but with my risk factors and the anxiety that's still intermittent, he is willing to deliver my son a few days earlier.

I answer without hesitation. "Yes, I would like to deliver my son on the thirteenth."

APRIL

↷ APRIL 1 *Thirty-six weeks*

I flip through the pages of *O, the Oprah Magazine* while bound to the machine that again monitors my son's heart rate. My legs are kicked up on a stool, and I now glance at the numbers after every few pages instead of every few paragraphs. There's no need to stare at the lines that map the crest of my contractions—there's only one or two, and with so much practice, I recognize the random pattern and faint intensity without looking at the graph. I do study my son's stats when I contract, an event that should make his heart rate bump up, and it does.

This nonstress test is routine, recommended by Dr. Mc-Conaughey as a precaution, not because I've had any symptoms of preterm labor the past few days. As we wait for our clean bill of health from Labor and Delivery, I stroke my belly and talk to my son—something I didn't dare do even a few months ago.

"*Are you bored with all of this, little guy?*" I stare down with affectionate eyes and quickly rub a small patch of my enormous stomach, as though I were mussing my son's hair. "*We get to meet you in twelve more days. Just twelve days!*"

I think about all the things we'll do together, long glorious walks with no regard for time or danger, the trips to the park where I'll push him in a swing while he kicks his toes and squeals with excitement, and the rocking chair where I'll stroke his hair under dim soft light, filling his head with tales of magic and adventure that will seep into his dreams after I nurse him to sleep.

I'll savor the pleasure of nursing my newborn son. Because Maddie was born so early, she had not yet developed a sucking reflex. She could only be fed through a feeding tube. I pumped milk every three hours around the clock, getting up through the night to make sure the hospital had enough milk for my tiny daughter. Making milk was of the utmost importance; it was the only tangible action I could take to care for my daughter. The pump made my nipples sore and crusted, and sometimes they bled, but I wouldn't stop. And because pumps aren't nearly as efficient as infants, my milk production was low, barely keeping up with her demand. On one of the nights when she was particularly hungry and the hospital was close to running out of breast milk, I pumped myself dry at two A.M. Jon jumped into the car and raced the container to the hospital, just in time to feed our thankfully ravenous and growing baby.

The nurse returns and inspects the data collected from the monitor. "He looks fine. Strong heart rate, and he was reactive when you contracted." She looks at me to see if her reassurances reached me.

I take a long, deep breath. I expected her report, but hearing the words from a medical professional will help when I'm worried tonight or tomorrow, when I'll replay the nurse's words in my head and chart his movement before I'm able to sleep.

"I really like Joshua. We could call him Josh." Jon sips his morning coffee while we lounge on the front porch sharing a lazy Sunday morning.

"I like it, too." I flip through the Styles section of the *New York Times.*

"So are we done? It is Joshua?"

I put down the paper and take in the emerging buds on the sturdy oak tree that anchors our front yard. "I don't know."

He looks mildly dismayed. "But you said you liked it."

"I do. And we know that Maddie likes it." I grin, thinking about the serious consideration she gave to each of our proposals. She deliberated for two days before agreeing that either would be acceptable.

He seems to ponder me for a moment. "Do you prefer Sam?"

"I don't know. I like it"—I nod in acknowledgment— "but I'm just not sure."

He sits back in his chair, but doesn't pick up the paper. Jon continues to glance toward me from the corner of his eye.

"Is it essential that we pick a name right now?" I meet his glance.

"No. I just don't understand why we can't."

"I just want to wait. That's all."

"Wait for what?"

"To see him. I don't want to name our son until I've seen him."

Jon now looks utterly confused.

"I love both of the names, but when I see him, he'll either look like a Josh, or look like a Sam. Then I'll know." I rest back in my chair, confident that he must now understand my desire to wait.

"But what does a Josh look like? And how exactly does a Josh look different from a Sam?"

"I can't explain it in those terms, Jon, but they just do. Can you trust me on this? Can we wait?"

"Sure, sure." He nods and picks up the crossword puzzle, but I still sense his poorly obscured need for closure. He is such a *man*.

APRIL 11 *Thirty-seven weeks and three days*

"What do you think of this one?" Ev holds up an off-white newborn sleeper with a tiny scalloped collar.

I reach out and touch the fabric. The solid cotton has an in-laid vertical stripe, but it still feels soft to the touch. I run my finger across the bottom of the scallops that border the collar and they easily bend. "That's a keeper. It should be comfortable against his skin."

Steve and Ev arrived last night to begin helping us prepare for our son. We have no nursery, never daring to be so confident. The only thing in the room with white walls and bare windows is Maddie's old baby bureau, just carried up from the basement. My mother-in-law carefully cleaned the inside of the drawers that haven't been used in years, stored after our move from California, awaiting the chance to be stuffed with clothes again.

"There's a little stain on this one, see?" Ev points to a spot on the leg of a yellow sleeper with tiny ducks sewn on the chest. "I bet I can wash that out. Do you want this one?"

Ev spent an hour sorting boxes in our stacked basement, locating all the boxes labeled "baby clothes: newborn" and "baby clothes: 6 months." "He'll grow so fast, you need to get them both ready," she advises.

We review the garments one at a time, rejecting the ones that look too stained or feel too harsh, scavenging the others that my son will wear after they've been washed and folded and tucked neatly into the wooden drawers of his baby bureau. After more than six years of storage, these barely worn jammies will finally get a second wave of use.

When we're done sorting, we have a few dozen items: sleepers and sweatpants, sweaters and jackets and T-shirts, and the collection of onesies that my girlfriends hand-painted at Maddie's social debut. I pick up the tiny shirts painted with teddy bears and flowers and rocking horses, note the initials painted in the corner of each shirt, and connect with each of these wondrous women who helped me celebrate my miraculous daughter as soon as her immune system was ready for a crowd—five months after her birth. The first few months after she came home from the hospital were spent guarding her from visitors, not risking exposure to common viruses that could overtake the underdeveloped immune response inherent in babies born so early. We risked few visitors beyond the nurse who made home visits to connect Maddie to needles and drip sacks to deliver immune-boosting drugs intravenously.

"I'll go wash these." Ev gathers up the tiny garments that we approved for her grandson's use and practically dances toward the laundry room as if she's boarding a plane for an exotic vacation. She is washing the newborn clothes that my son will wear when I take him for walks and errands, and when friends come to meet him, his parents able to indulge in the joys of a new infant instead of standing sentry against the common viruses that full-term babies can usually handle. When she returns, two piles of rejected items remain on the floor: too soiled, and too girly.

"I knew I couldn't reuse the dresses with a boy, but I had no idea I pinked out so early with Maddie." We laugh about the vibrantly colored pile of every shade of pink in dresses and skirts and sleepers and sweaters.

"What should I do with these?" Ev points to the piles. We decide to donate the items that look too stained after one last spin in the washer. "And the others?" She looks at the pile of perfectly reusable baby girl clothes.

I glance through the items, remembering Maddie's first stroll when I bundled her in the pink sweater with the silver buttons shaped like little teapots, and the pink knit dress with the matching bloomers that she wore to her first dinner out with me and Jon, months after her early arrival. My thoughts slip back to the daughter I lost, and I wonder how she would have looked bundled up in these soft pink sweaters and plush knit hats. "Can you please put those back in the storage boxes for the basement?"

Ev looks confused by my decision, but she collects the girl clothes and heads downstairs.

~ ~ ~

Maddie beams as she walks through the front door with my father-in-law. She sticks out her chest and hides something behind her back.

"Where have you two been?" I can only imagine the

indulgences Steve has served up to my daughter while they were out. He takes her to Chuck E. Cheese's for endless games, to toy stores to pillage shelves, and to candy stores from which she returns with a month's worth of desserts. Even as grandparents go, he's a real pushover.

"We were at the hospital," she says.

"There was something she had to get. She's been asking me to take her from the moment we got here yesterday." Steve looks pleased, proud.

Maddie grins as she pulls the plush blue bunny from behind her back. "It's for my baby brother. I wanted to be the first one to get him a present."

She hands me the bunny, so soft it melts under my fingers, with ears that flop across its dark stitched eyes and little plastic nose. Sewn across the bunny's white chest are the words *It's a boy.* Maddie explains that she saw it in the hospital gift shop on one of the trips when Daddy took her exploring while I spoke to the doctor. "I was afraid they might run out of blue ones," she says, "so I had Poppop take me today."

"Good thinking." I fold my thoughtful daughter into my arms and bury my face in her golden-red curls. "He's awfully lucky to have a big sister like you."

She looks pleased.

I look toward Steve and notice that he also holds something sheepishly behind his back. His eyes dart before he reveals the pink bunny. "It just didn't seem fair. You can't have one grandchild get a present and not the other."

I grin at his mindful violation of our house rules. Steve and Ev were spoiling Maddie with so many presents that we insisted their gifts be limited to birthdays and holidays.

"What's a more special occasion than this?" he pleads.

"You're absolutely right. Thank you. I can see why you had to get that for her." I catch Maddie's eye and give her a wink.

APRIL 12 *Thirty-seven weeks and four days*

"I feel this one." I clutch my stomach as the monitor graphs the cresting pain from my contraction. I called Dr. McConaughey when I woke up this morning with rhythmic back pain that is now accompanied by contractions more forceful than any of the other episodes.

Dr. Stiller, the ER doctor I saw in February, examines the scroll of graph paper after more than an hour of monitoring. "That one was more intense, but still moderate," she reports as I grasp the arms of the recliner. I've had several contractions over the past hour or so. My uterus stiffens and the pain is sufficient to take my breath until the pain subsides.

"Based on what I see, I think you're in the early stages of labor," she says.

I nod, watching my son's heart rate on the machine, confirmation that he is not in distress, that he is fine. The numbers that flash on the monitor chase away the fear that still lingers, even at this late stage of pregnancy. "I'm scheduled to deliver tomorrow. The C-section is set for nine o'clock."

She holds her fist to her lips before surveying the monitoring results again. "You have two choices here. You can try to wait it out until tomorrow, or we can take you in right now for an emergency C-section."

I suppose I shouldn't be, but I'm surprised by her response. After so many incidents of monitoring followed by discharge to "watchfully wait" at home, I'm not sure what to say; I haven't practiced this part before. "Can Dr. McConaughey do the C-section today?"

"No. If we do it now, I will deliver your son. If you want Dr. McConaughey to deliver, you'll have to hold out until tomorrow morning."

"What do you think my chances are of making it until tomorrow?"

She looks up as if calculating on a whiteboard in her head. "Maybe fifty percent. If you go home, I think you're likely to be back sometime tonight."

She leaves to give me a moment to consider my options. I grab my cell to give Jon a chance to weigh in. I update him on my contractions, and the chance that our choice may not matter.

"So this is really it?" His voice is rife with excitement and anxiety.

"It was going to be 'it' tomorrow, anyway. But yes, it could be today." I glance at my son's numbers, his strong, regular heart rate dampening the embers of my angst.

"What do you want to do?" Jon waits.

We discuss all the rational points: our close proximity to the hospital, the monitoring that confirms he's okay for now, our strong trust in Dr. McConaughey.

But there's something beyond rational thought that dances through my mind; the beauty and redemption of faith flows through my body in tingling impulses that unbind the knots of fear. After so much tragedy, when my spirit limped and existed only as a shadow, I must now decide where to take the last step in this pregnancy: I can step toward fear, or I can step toward faith.

I think about the months that followed Maddie's birth, how she spent nearly two months in an NICU, her discharge followed by months of hypervigilance when I expected her to stop breathing at any moment, as I'd seen in the NICU. And after she'd been home for ten days, she did. Her body went limp and her eyes rolled back as she sat in her car seat. I screamed and grabbed her out, jostled her back to consciousness just as I'd seen the nurses do. Jon and I raced back to the hospital where she was admitted for overnight observation, where we both sat by her crib, staring at the monitors until dawn. I spent the first year of her life tortured by these memories, fearing that she could die at any moment, casting a flashlight toward her chest a dozen times every night to make sure she was breathing.

I don't want to spend the first year of my son's life gripped with fear. I want to know the freedom of carefree strolls down the street, and putting him down for a nap without wondering whether he'll wake up. I want the peace, the joy, the redemption of belief.

"Jon, if it doesn't make you uncomfortable, I think I want to go home."

~ ~ ~

"We're ready for you to come down." Jon's voice floats up the stairs to my bed where I've rested since getting home. Dr. Stiller said I should lie down to have the best chance of making it until the morning, but I've given myself permission to have one last dinner as a pregnant woman, with my family. I rise from my bed, what I now realize has been the outermost womb for my son.

Dinner is already plated and waiting when I get to the dining room table. Jon and Steve asked what I wanted for my last dinner, and then gathered the finest ingredients to assemble a decadent version of my request: cheeseburgers. Really good cheeseburgers.

The table is set with glistening white plates and a centerpiece of red and yellow Gerbera daisies with layers of petals that converge into their soft dark pistils. The air is filled with the excitement of a party or a holiday, and we all bounce into our chairs as chatter floats through the room. I bite into the seeded bun that lightly crunches when my teeth break through the toasted edges, sinking into grilled onions and thick ground sirloin that dribbles juice down my chin.

"This is absolutely delicious." I nod appreciatively toward my chefs, savoring the texture and flavors of this perfect creation. We feast on burgers and oven roasted potatoes tossed in olive oil and rosemary. When the last bite is gone, Ev heads to the kitchen for chocolate chip cookies, still warm from the oven.

"Can I give her the present yet?" Maddie looks at Jon as though she may burst. He nods and she runs from the room, returning with a slick white box bound with a red satin ribbon. Maddie is practically jumping out of her skin for me to open it.

"Do you want to open it for me?" I ask.

She seizes the chance, ripping the ribbon and holding up a tiny, backless, red summer dress.

"Maddie, it's beautiful." I hold up the dress, admiring the color and praising her thoughtfulness as I glimpse the size six tag, a milestone that seems unachievable for this body that now engulfs the chair. "You didn't have to get Mommy a present, sweetie. But this was so nice of you."

"I know I didn't. But you've worked so hard to have this baby, you deserve special treatment." She looks serious, mature. I look around the room wondering which set of adult lips she heard this from. "Go put it on," she says.

"Oh . . . well . . ." I turn the dress and examine it from all sides, imagining the seams bursting as I try to stuff all of my pregnant-with-fifty-extra-pounds self into this distant possibility. "I don't think it would fit just yet, sweetie. But Mommy can't wait to wear it after I lose the baby weight." I grab Maddie for a huge hug, silently wondering whether she'll grow into the dress before I thin down for it.

~ ~ ~

"When was the last contraction?" Jon slips on pajama bottoms as he sizes me up from his closet. I lie in our sleigh bed, propped up with pillows, flipping through the pages of fashion magazines that Ev bought for mindless distraction.

"I haven't felt one in a while. At least twenty minutes or so." The unmarked paper and pencil are perched on my nightstand, waiting to chart the pains if they become more frequent or more intense. The pains have eased a bit since I spent the afternoon in bed, only venturing downstairs for a quick dinner before tucking back in.

"Do you think we'll make it all night?" Jon climbs into bed like a kid going on his first sleepover. I grin at my husband, sometimes so adolescent despite the gray hairs that now pepper his temples and the fine lines around green eyes that still glisten when he looks at me.

I shrug my shoulders while I flip through the pages, stopping at an Armani ad where a pencil-legged model wears high heels and a fluted white miniskirt with dark trim. She strides with the confidence of youth and style, looking like a woman who has never even changed a diaper, much less staggered for six years fighting for the privilege to do so. I glance down at my body that bulges under the blankets, touch my hair that hasn't been cut in nine months, and peer toward the closet where my new red dress hangs among the baggy jeans and sweats that have been my casual wardrobe for years. I remember when I wore short skirts and high heels, when I actually tried to look current and sexy and reasonably youthful.

I start stammering to Jon about how awful I look, how I can't wait to finally be done with pregnancies and grief and get my body back, how I long for the indulgence of a carefree shopping trip instead of spending every spare moment reading research studies and medical books. Jon listens patiently to my admissions. "And I'm starting here, with these." I pull back the blankets and crunch the cotton fabric of my maternity sweats, just like the ones I wear to bed when I'm not pregnant, only bigger. "As soon as I lose the baby belly, I'm going straight out to buy silk nighties."

Jon stares at me, perplexed. Then he speaks. "When did you stop wearing silk to bed?"

My mouth drops. I stare in disbelief at the husband who gazes at me with eyes so taken they must only see the bride of ten years ago. He reaches over and caresses my face before leaning in for a long, delicate kiss. I run my fingers through his hair, now reveling in his failure to clearly see what's right before his eyes.

APRIL 13 *Thirty-seven weeks and five days*

"Are you nervous?" Jon stands by my bed just before nine A.M., holding my hand. The anesthesiologist has left after inserting the spinal. I lie on the gurney, waiting to be wheeled into the operating room where we'll meet our son in moments.

"A little." A surgical knife is about to be sliced through my abdomen; the thought is a bit unsettling. But I've been through the procedure once, with Maddie, so I know what to expect. And today, I have faith.

"Can you believe we're about to meet our son?" My voice trembles with excitement as I squeeze Jon's hand. He looks back with a goofy smile.

"We've built our family. After all of it, we'll finally be a family of four." He closes his lips tightly and lowers his head.

I nod, feeling fortunate and blessed to be here awaiting my son's arrival. But I also can't help but think of my other children, the ones who never came home. I imagine them somehow knowing, sharing our joy. "We were almost a family of five. Do you remember when Dr. D told us we were having twins?"

Jon's face tells me that we're both looking back and connecting to the shock and joy of that moment. We had planned for two children, but the idea of three quickly grew on us, quickly felt right. We both slip into a moment of longing for the family we almost had.

"I know we're lucky—we're about to have a son. But there's a part of me that feels . . . well . . . cheated." Jon bites his lip. "I get that there are no guarantees, but I still feel like we were supposed to have three kids, like our family was shorted."

"Me too. I will cherish my two children, but if things were different, we'd have more."

We look at each other in silence, knowing what the other is thinking.

"Jon, I don't know that I could ever be pregnant again. But there is a part of me—"

"Are you having doubts about the tubal ligation?"

"Yes. And no. It would be insane for me to get pregnant again. Absolutely insane." I shake my head.

"Completely nuts."

"Completely."

"But you do have some doubt?"

I don't know if it's the euphoria of the moment, the hope that seems so undefeatable in the moments just before birth, or my dream of a minivan filled with children, but at this moment, I do have doubt about the tubal. "A sliver."

"Then we shouldn't do it. Darci, it's permanent. We could never have another baby."

Dr. McConaughey walks in for one final check before we go in for the C-section. He smiles from ear to ear. "I am so happy to see you here."

Jon and I both chuckle.

"There's one last paperwork detail before we get started. I need you to sign the consent forms for the C-section and the tubal ligation."

I look toward Jon while my sliver of doubt makes tiny incisions into my resolve.

"Dr. McConaughey, we've changed our minds about the tubal. I don't want the tubal ligation."

~ ~ ~

"The cerclage is out." Dr. McConaughey leans over the blue tent that blocks the view below my shoulders. From the dwindling cervix and recurring funneling that appeared throughout my pregnancy, I know that without these few stitches around a synthetic band that held my cervix closed, I would have lost my son; if I had not sought this treatment that many physicians would not offer until three or more later losses—the recommended medical standard to warrant cerclage—I would not be on this table today. "Let's get her positioned for the C-section," the doctor instructs.

People tug at my legs and shift my body down. I can feel nothing below my chest. I look up at Jon with excitement and apprehension. He squeezes my shoulder, aware that I'm checking in, but quickly turns his attention back to the other end of the table.

"I'll start the C-section now." Dr. McConaughey speaks with me to confirm my pain-free state before metal instruments chink. I think he has made the first incision because Jon's face begins to contort where he stands above me, watching the procedure. When his face starts to whiten, I know the procedure is progressing further inward.

"Okay. You are open and clamped off. I'm going to rupture the membranes."

Jon leans forward, tentatively, like opening a closet door without being certain what's inside. His face is mildly aghast. The medical team chatters while they go through these routine motions, but their voices twinge with anticipation. Despite how common this scene must be at the hospital, I sense they still look forward to unveiling children to the world.

"We need to push the baby out by maneuvering your lower abdomen. You will feel some pressure." Dr. McConaughey then asks the group if they're ready.

Whomp. The doctors and nurses push and squeeze my stomach, pulling so hard that my body lifts off the table and smacks back down. *Whomp.* They lift again. This part certainly is new; with Maddie, the doctor made a quick incision and lifted her right out. I had no idea that full-term babies were adhered with some sort of Super Glue, and that a full-term C-section resembled a WWE throwdown.

I'm not sure exactly how all this looks, but Jon is starting to turn his face away. I don't know if it's the surprise of how physical the delivery is, or the anticipation of seeing our son, but I suddenly feel anxious. Is he supposed to be stuck so tightly? Are they having a problem? My God, is our son all right?

I start to work myself into a dither. Then I see him. Every sound and motion in the room evaporates as I stare, silent, surreal, at our son.

Dr. McConaughey beams as he holds this cherished prize with two gloved hands over the edges of my tent. "Here's your boy."

Our son doesn't cry. He puckers his face and tries to orient his batting eyes to the first rays of light ever seen. His body is red and covered with thick clear goo that darkens the lonely wisps of hair matted to his head. He kicks his legs and rotates his arms in stiff motions, like a senior in an exercise class. Our little man takes in the new world just thrust upon him like a true New Englander, with strong resolve.

I reach out and touch him, safe, here, his skin so soft I draw my fingers back in fear that their relative coarseness may cause him pain. My eyes fill with awe as past fears dissolve and all the hope and possibility of the future wiggles before me.

I grab Jon's hand and squeeze it before looking back at Dr. McConaughey. "Sam. Our son's name is Sam."

Jon looks at me on the table and nods before shielding his eyes to hide his tears.

My chin quivers. We actually made it, past the constant danger that threatened to preclude this moment, threatened to steal this wondrous child that will grow up and strive to somehow make the world better. We now stare in near disbelief at the miracle that stretches and squirms and puckers before us, and today, we have both seen grace.

~ ~ ~

The aftermath of the anesthesia tries to lull me to sleep as I watch Maddie hold Sam against her chest. He is tightly swaddled in white flannel hospital blankets and sleeps peacefully, held securely in his sister's arms. Maddie wears a smile that's wide and unyielding, as though her two ponytails have permanently cinched her lips in an elated expression. Ev stands sentry, checking Maddie's arms every few minutes to ensure that Sam is properly supported.

I can barely keep my eyes open, but after waiting so long to see my son, safe and healthy, and my daughter, glowing in the radiance from new life, I can't miss even a moment.

"Do you need to sleep?" Jon walks over and strokes my hair, apparently noticing my eyelids growing heavier.

"No, I don't want him to be alone." I gaze at our son. *Our son.* "Besides, I'm not that tired," I lie.

"We could take him to the nursery and sit with him there," Jon offers. "He wouldn't be alone."

"No. I don't want him out of my room. But maybe I will take just a little nap." Jon hands me the sleeping mask I brought from home. I glance around my room where Maddie, Ev, and Steve all take turns with Jon to hold the newest member of the Klein family. "Jon," I mumble, "you'll make sure that Maddie's arms don't get too tired, that he's properly supported?"

"Yes."

"And his airway needs to be clear. Make sure Sam's neck isn't crunched up so that his throat gets compressed."

"I understand." Jon strokes my arm. "Sam is safe. You can go to sleep."

I nod, then take one last glance at my tiny miracle before slipping on the velvet mask and drifting off.

~ APRIL 15

"He is absolutely beautiful." Mary sits in the recliner of my hospital room holding Sam while he sleeps. She looks at him with a reverence and contentment usually confined to new moms.

"I wish you could see him with his eyes open. They're such a deep blue." Warmth trickles through my chest as I talk about the newest love in my life.

Mary nods as she nestles Sam in the recliner, swaying back and forth in even motions, whispering to him how happy we all are that he's here.

I start to unpack the Thai food that Mary brought for lunch, placing white take-out cartons on the rolling tray by my bed.

"I'll do that," she says, rising slowly with Sam still in her arms.

"No. I'd like to serve you for a change. Besides, look how happy he is."

She slides back down, picking up the whispered promises and lulling motions right where she left off. I open the first box, where vegetable spring rolls lie on a bed of julienned carrots and alfalfa sprouts with pert green blossoms. I grab the next container and inhale peanuts mixed with hints of tamarind and fish sauce, opening the top to see pad thai with slivers of scallions and flat glistening noodles. Remarkably for two women at lunch, a third container lurks in the bottom of the bag. The familiar scent of chilies and coriander and cumin drifts up as I lift the last dish from the bag: my favorite, red curry chicken.

"This is decadent." I grin while assembling two plates, mine still much fuller than Mary's. "I know I'll have to start cutting back on the food a little, but I'm still healing. And I need to make milk." I glance at my still-robust body, reduced by a mere ten pounds after delivery.

"Yes. Still healing—and you should enjoy." Mary eases Sam into the crib that stays in my room day and night. She grabs her plate while we go through the book of baby stores around Boston. "Everything from cribs to paint to sleepers, it's all in here," she says.

I glance through the room and survey my blessings, a healthy sleeping son and a deep new friendship forged in only months, as my style guide flips through the pages, providing personal reviews of the stores and products. I look at the pages and envision a colorful nursery where my baby will sleep and play and jump, and his mother will look on in wonder.

APRIL 17

We glide into our driveway and Jon shifts the van into park. We look up at the tall blue house shrouded by old growth oaks and pines that reach toward a pristine azure sky. In the back our precious cargo waits, a now six-year-old girl who can't stop smiling, and a son who seems to deeply contemplate his first ride in a car.

"I'll carry him in." Jon releases the infant car seat from the base and lifts Sam with the care reserved for a jeweled crown resting atop a plush pillow. I tuck soft blankets tightly around his sides and adjust his white cap, careful to protect him from the cool winds of spring in New England. We saunter up our stone stairs as Maddie races past, eager to tell Nanny and Poppop that we're home. They open the front door before she gets to the last step.

"Look who's home." Steve stares where we all stare, at the little bundled miracle with blue eyes that rove the room, completely unaware of his stature in the house.

Jon eases the car seat to the floor, where Sam rests for the first time in his home.

I gaze at our son and start to dissolve. The fears and perils barely dodged over the past nine months swirl through my head while I study this miracle that nearly wasn't ours. The enormity of what we went through feels crushing as I consider how different my life could be at this moment, how different it was, coming home from the hospital nearly two years ago, without the children I'd given birth to.

I weep, shaken by how terrifyingly close I came to losing my son on so many occasions, and overwhelmed by the memory of what was lost, a child at thirteen weeks, another at eight weeks, twins at twenty weeks. These children were never carried so preciously into their new home, this moment never shared with our other beloved babies.

Jon and I clutch each other and he starts to sob.

"Why are they crying?" Maddie asks Steve.

"Tears of joy, Maddie. They're happy." He pulls her close and reassures her.

Jon and I finally loosen our grip and sit on the floor, one on each side of Sam's car seat. I peel back the blankets and run my finger down his leg covered by the cushy white jumper that Ev picked up for his journey home. Jon gently grasps Sam's tiny fingers, mystified by their very existence. I stroke Sam's cheek in amazement, anticipating the contours on the face already traced hundreds of times in slow, careful motions. I detach the harness and fold our son into my arms.

"Sam, this is your home. We've all been so eager for you to get here." My voice is just above a whisper as I press my lips against his forehead. "You'll be very happy here. We promise."

WHAT EVERY WOMAN
SHOULD KNOW ABOUT
PREGNANCY LOSS

I am not a doctor. I am a woman who became determined to have another baby, and after realizing that obstetric guidelines do little to diagnose pregnancy loss, I knew I had to do my own research. Luckily, I'm a career market researcher with a master's from the University of Chicago. My background allowed me to critically evaluate the reliability of many research studies and interview specialists across the country for greater insight into pregnancy loss. After deep exploration, I concluded that obstetrics is rich with controversy. The field often lacks certainty, primarily due to a dearth of research dollars and a society that enables miscarriage by accepting these tragedies as unfortunate and unavoidable, without questioning whether we can do better.

If you are a woman who experiences the tragedy of miscarriage, you'll have to decide whether to demand testing after loss.

As you make your decision, please consider the issues that my research uncovered.

Miscarriage is a common problem.

Many women experience the tragedy of miscarriage, but the exact number is unknown. States are not required to report information on pregnancy losses prior to twenty weeks gestation, and thus only estimates are available.

Researchers estimate that between 2.3 million and 5.4 million miscarriages occur in the United States every year—30 to 50 percent of all pregnancies.[28] These estimates include preclinical losses, defined as pregnancies lost before six weeks gestation.

The most commonly reported estimates of pregnancy loss understate the problem by failing to include preclinical losses, thought to account for at least half of all miscarriages.[29] The U.S. National Vital Statistics Report estimates that approximately one million *clinically diagnosed* pregnancies are lost every year;[30] the American College of Obstetricians and Gynecologists (ACOG), which sets the standards for obstetric care, reports that 10 to 15 percent of *clinically diagnosed* pregnancies end in loss.[31] So according to official statistics, both literally and figuratively, babies lost before six weeks gestation simply do not count.

No group disputes that the incidence of miscarriage is increasing. As more women delay childbearing, often attempting pregnancy after age thirty-five when careers and relationships are more established, the chance of miscarriage rises to 70 percent.[32]

During the past decade, a likely *20 million* women in the United States alone have endured the physical pain and emotional anguish of miscarriage. Yet even with the pervasiveness of this problem, the medical community treats miscarriage as a mere rite of passage, not a legitimate medical condition that warrants diagnostic testing and preventive treatment.

ACOG guidelines say that women should not be tested for causes of pregnancy loss until *multiple consecutive losses* have occurred, and even then, an investigation often doesn't happen unless demanded by the patient.

Doctors do not routinely test for causes of miscarriage. Traditional medical guidelines stated that women must endure *three or more consecutive* pregnancy losses before physicians consider any diagnostic testing. As of 2001, the guidelines were revised to *two or more consecutive* losses,[33] but many obstetricians focus on the *or more* instead of the *two*, failing to offer testing after a second loss.

High-risk obstetricians regularly see women who have never been offered testing, even after three, four, or five losses. One physician I spoke with had a patient with twelve prior losses, no investigations ever completed. Even after multiple losses, many women will not be tested unless they demand it, and most women simply don't know to ask.

Because testing guidelines require that losses be *consecutive* to matter, the rule ignores a central truth of obstetrics: Few conditions that can cause pregnancy loss actually do so in each and every pregnancy; many obstetric disorders strike only sporadically. Under the current guideline, women with one successful pregnancy interspersed between two losses do not warrant testing.

ACOG testing guidelines also have an inherent, offensive implication: that lost babies are interchangeable. Their reasoning says that testing is unwarranted before multiple losses because when women keep trying, they will likely succeed the next time. But what about the miscarriages that were lost? What about the *hundreds of thousands* of miscarriages that occur in this country each year that could have been prevented if undiscovered disorders were diagnosed and treated? Women grieved these miscarriages. Each one would have been a daughter or a son. To these grieving families, these babies mattered.

Instead of being offered testing after pregnancy loss, women are usually quoted questionable statistics and told simply to "keep trying."
After multiple losses, women are told that their odds of having a baby without any testing or intervention are high, but much controversy exists about whether this is actually true.

ACOG says that after two consecutive miscarriages, only 30 percent of women will lose the next pregnancy, and after three consecutive miscarriages, just 33 percent will lose their next baby.[34] These estimates are primarily based on studies from decades ago, before practitioners had the technology to reliably detect pregnancies lost before six weeks. Because at least 50 percent of miscarriages happen before six weeks,[35] these studies underreported the rate of pregnancy loss.

Many high-risk specialists believe the risk of miscarriage after two losses is 40 percent, and after three losses the chance climbs to 60 percent,[36] much higher than ACOG's projections. These practitioners base their belief on multiple studies as well as the wisdom of their own practices, in which they deliver care that goes well beyond ACOG standards to successfully treat patients after multiple tragedies.

Ultimately, there are no definitive, reliable studies to provide a clear answer to the chance of yet another miscarriage, but one thing is clear: With odds so questionable, many women would choose testing, if only someone gave them a choice to make.

Women are told that most losses are due to fetal chromosome abnormalities, but the likelihood that chromosome errors caused a miscarriage is low when a baby developed beyond ten weeks gestation, or when the mother is younger than thirty years old.
The most common cause of miscarriage is fetal chromosome abnormalities. These aberrations are random and untreatable and account for half of all losses. Because this is such a frequent cause of miscarriage, doctors often assume this is the cause of loss without considering the baby's gestational age at the time of loss or the mother's age, two factors that significantly change the likelihood of these abnormalities.

As gestational age of the pregnancy increases, the likelihood of chromosome abnormalities decreases. For miscarriages before six weeks gestation, 70 percent are believed to be caused by chromosomal abnormalities; between six and ten weeks, 50 percent; and after ten weeks, a mere 5 percent.[37] Despite the low likelihood that chromosomal errors are the cause of losses after ten weeks, women with one later miscarriage are virtually never offered any testing.

Note that these statistics apply to the time when the pregnancy stopped developing, not the time when bleeding started and the pregnancy begins to be expelled. In some cases a woman's body may take weeks to realize that her developing baby has died, and thus the first signs of miscarriage may not appear until several weeks after the date of the actual loss—deemed by the medical world as the "time of demise." Physicians can estimate the time of demise with an ultrasound, but this approximation can be off by several weeks.

The likelihood of errant chromosomes also varies with the mother's age. For women under age twenty-five, only 36 percent of losses are found to be abnormal; for women age thirty-five to thirty-nine, 68 percent of losses are abnormal.[38] Despite the differing age-related probabilities of chromosome abnormalities, many physicians still chalk up losses suffered by younger women to "acts of nature."

Note that when testing confirms bad chromosomes, the medical community considers the loss "explained," and for most women this is the only culprit; however, this test does not rule out the presence of other medical conditions that could claim future pregnancies. Although multiple losses can be caused exclusively by errant chromosomes, patients who continue to lose pregnancies should consider further testing.

After miscarriage, testing for chromosome abnormalities is critical. The results definitively separate women into two groups: those whose loss was caused by chance, and those who need further testing to protect future pregnancies.

Women should demand chromosome analysis after any suspicious pregnancy loss.
According to one recently published study, women should ask for chromosome analysis of the lost miscarriage (1) for any first loss that developed beyond ten weeks gestation or (2) any second or subsequent miscarriage, regardless of the gestational age of the lost baby.[39] Under either of these conditions, the loss is suspicious because of the diminished probability of fetal chromosome errors.

This recommendation is highly controversial. Few obstetricians ever test after a first loss, regardless of the gestational age at the time of loss. Most defend their decision by quoting ACOG guidelines that discourage testing until two or more consecutive losses; others say that insurance companies will not pay for the test until there are a minimum of two consecutive losses.

But shouldn't patients be involved in this decision? If an insurer refuses to pay, the patient can fight with the insurer, or pay out of pocket. I'm told that the test costs between $600 and $800, and that is a lot of money. But if this is really about money, shouldn't the patient be given a choice about whether to do the test?

While the study I've cited recommends testing for any second or subsequent loss, as well as first miscarriages beyond ten weeks, I would encourage women to consider chromosomal testing for any first loss after six weeks. For losses between six and ten weeks, the odds are high that fetal chromosomes were normal, and many of these women have an underlying disorder that could claim future pregnancies without treatment.

Some specialists also advise that women seek chromosome analysis after any pregnancy loss that used assisted reproductive technology, such as in vitro fertilization (IVF) and especially after repeated IVF failures.

When chromosome testing is requested after a loss, 91 percent of women get a conclusive result when the patient undergoes a D&C to collect a fetal sample for testing. Patients are sometimes advised to collect a sample by expectant management—meaning the patient forgoes a D&C and collects sanitary pads and any passed tissue at home, taking this material to her doctor for testing. When patients use expectant management, only 66 percent will get a conclusive result about the lost baby's chromosomes.[40]

Note that some couples do get inconclusive results after fetal chromosome testing. *Inconclusive* means that the chromosomes could not be effectively cultured for analysis, often because of contamination of the sample, and thus the chromosomal status of the miscarriage remains unknown. This was a far more common occurrence in years past, but improvements in testing methodologies have greatly increased the reliability of this test.[41] Also, conclusive results are more likely when the sample is fresh, and thus women should send fetal tissue for testing as soon as possible.

When considering how best to collect tissue for testing, patients should speak with their physicians about any personal risk factors that should be considered when making their choice. Some physicians believe that a D&C can create uterine scar tissue, which may impair future pregnancies.

After chromosomally normal pregnancies are lost, a thorough evaluation can reveal a treatable cause in the majority of cases.

A rigorous study published more than a decade ago found that 60 percent of women who lost a chromosomally normal pregnancy had a treatable but undiagnosed condition.[42] Advances made over the past decade in reproductive immunology are known to boost this number even higher, possibly to 80 percent.[43] Because some disorders cause pregnancy loss only sporadically, a portion of these women could have a successful pregnancy without treatment. Others will continue to miscarry if not diagnosed and treated.

When seeking testing after loss, it's important to know exactly what tests are being administered. The depth of evaluation can vary from doctor to doctor. ACOG guidelines from 2001 recommend only three tests after early (before fifteen weeks) recurrent pregnancy loss, and they project that 50 to 75 percent of couples will find no treatable cause after undergoing this narrow band of tests.[44] Mainstream doctors who follow these guidelines will likely administer fewer diagnostic tests than specialists and other obstetricians who explore a wider range of causes.

When diagnostic testing is completed, the 2001 ACOG guidelines recommend the following evaluations for early recurrent pregnancy loss:

- Lupus anticoagulant and anticardiolipin antibodies to test for antiphospholipid syndrome
- Parental balanced chromosome abnormalities
- Uterine abnormalities

A recently published paper argues that if the following three additional evaluations were added to ACOG's standard evaluation, significantly more women would receive a diagnosis:

- Prolactin levels to test for luteal phase defect
- TSH to evaluate thyroid function
- Factor V Leiden mutation[45]

If no answers are found after these tests, or if patients desire a deeper investigation, many additional evaluations can be sought through your obstetrician, or at facilities that specialize in treating recurrent pregnancy loss. At these university centers and clinics, patients are usually evaluated for an extended set of possible causes—some that are extremely rare, and others that are supported by limited or developing evidence, including additional inherited thrombophilias beyond Factor V Leiden, and other immunological disorders. Regardless of where care is sought, it is critical to know which tests have been completed and, if further diagnosis is sought, to seek out a qualified special-ist who will take the time to explain which additional evalua-tions should be completed.

In the reference section in the back of this book, I've listed several obstetric organizations whose members specialize in di-agnosing, treating, and preventing pregnancy loss. These organi-zations refer patients to specialists in their geographic area. Most couples find success with these maternal-fetal medicine, en-docrinology, and immunology specialists who deliver care that far exceeds recommended standards.

Note that the tests just discussed refer to pregnancies lost at the earlier stages of gestation. While these evaluations may be relevant for losses that occurred in the second or third trimester, additional factors, such as cervical incompetence and many oth-ers, should be considered when diagnosing later losses.

At least 700,000 pregnancies succumb to treatable disorders every year.

Because 60 percent of women who lose chromosomally normal pregnancies have an undiagnosed but treatable disorder, 700,000 babies are lost each year to conditions that could have been treated if diagnosed. I believe this is a conservative estimate. We know that advances in reproductive immunology increase the number of diagnosable women beyond 60 percent, but without more research, we can't be certain exactly how much.

Sadly, none of these babies will ever be saved; some disor-ders have no symptoms before the first pregnancy loss. But if women were not forced to endure multiple losses before being tested, if fetal chromosomal analysis were offered after every suspicious miscarriage—any first loss after six weeks, and any second or subsequent loss, regardless of gestational age—

disorders could be detected and treated before so many lives were needlessly lost.

Even more babies could be saved if testing were appropriately expanded for inherited thrombophilias, especially mutations such as Factor V Leiden, which strong evidence links to pregnancy loss. These mutations might be flagged before even one pregnancy loss in some women if obstetricians gathered the patient's family history of pregnancy loss. While most obstetricians ask about family medical events such as heart attacks and stroke and diabetes, information that is certainly relevant, I've seen few new-patient intake forms that ask about the family history of pregnancy loss. When a woman's mother or sister has endured multiple miscarriages, especially if the losses were in the second or third trimester, inherited thrombophilias such as Factor V Leiden should be suspected and tested for. And if any patient has a history of blood clots, these evaluations should be completed.

More aggressive monitoring for indicators of preterm labor would also prevent many losses. Some hospitals do this by routinely taking a cervical measurement as part of any Level II ultrasound, a specialized scan that most women get between sixteen and twenty weeks gestation. This is simply standard procedure at some hospitals, but not all. Also, any woman who has experienced a loss in the second or third trimester should ask her doctor about serial cervical measurements during subsequent pregnancies. Standard guidelines leave obstetricians tremendous discretion about whether to take cervical measurements, only recommending this step after *two or more* late losses that are considered unexplained, meaning another cause of loss was not established. If more women received regular measurements after a single late loss, many who have already known the horror of late loss would be spared the tragedy of losing another child.

Inherited thrombophilias are a suspected cause of pregnancy loss.

Thrombophilia is the tendency to form blood clots. Healthy bodies continually form and then break down blood clots. With thrombophilia, the body's ability to dissolve clots is impaired. Thrombophilia can develop in adults, a condition known as acquired thrombophilia, or it can result from a gene mutation, a condition known as inherited thrombophilia.

Thrombophilia can cause fetal complications during pregnancy when blood clots travel to the placenta or the umbilical cord. These clots can block the flow of nutrients to the developing baby, leading to pregnancy loss or complications such as fetal growth retardation. In several studies, some thrombotic mutations have also been linked to other pregnancy complications, such as preeclampsia and placental abruption. To date, seven inherited thrombophilias have been identified. Among the more common are Factor V Leiden, prothrombin gene mutation, and protein S deficiency, thought to affect 6 percent, 4 to 13 percent, and 5 to 8 percent of women, respectively. The presence of these mutations has been associated with an increased risk of pregnancy loss in multiple studies,[46] but the strength of the evidence varies for each of the specific seven mutations. Some physicians feel strongly that evidence warrants treating any of these seven mutations; other physicians choose to treat none of them.

ACOG describes the role of all inherited thrombophilias in pregnancy loss as "controversial." Its guidelines say that physicians should not test for inherited thrombophilias as part of an early recurrent pregnancy loss evaluation, but such testing should be considered only for cases of late loss when no other cause can be found.[47]

Thorough loss evaluations usually reveal *several possible causes* of loss instead of *one definite culprit*—yet another illustration of the uncertainty in obstetrics. But with ACOG's stance on inherited thrombophilias as a test of last resort, obstetricians who strictly follow guidelines rarely administer this test, and thus their patients remain unaware of mutations that may cause future losses and are given no choice about treatment.

Strong evidence links Factor V Leiden to recurrent pregnancy loss.

Although the strength of evidence linking all inherited thrombophilias to suspicious pregnancy loss varies, the case for Factor V Leiden is exceptionally strong, and a growing number of physicians test for Factor V Leiden after a suspicious loss. Some ten million women carry this mutation. Fourteen case-controlled studies have found a higher prevalence of this mutation in women with unexplained recurrent pregnancy loss.[48] A large analysis of three thousand women found that carriers of this mutation have twice the risk of noncarriers for first-trimester loss, but nearly eight times the risk for late (after thirteen weeks) recurrent fetal loss.[49] And in one frequently cited study linking Factor V Leiden with recurrent pregnancy loss, only 37 percent of women with the mutation had a live birth; among the control group without the mutation, 69 percent had a live birth.[50] Despite research that establishes higher loss rates when Factor V Leiden is present, existing guidelines do not differentiate Factor V Leiden from other inherited thrombophilias, thus instructing doctors to rarely check for this mutation.

If physicians diagnose Factor V Leiden or other inherited thrombophilias, patients can be treated with a daily injection of an anticoagulant (heparin) and low-dose aspirin. To date, no randomized clinical trial—the gold standard in research—has been performed to verify the efficacy of heparin for inherited thrombophilias, but some studies strongly indicate that treatment can prevent losses. In the only controlled (using an untreated group for comparison) treatment study of women with the Factor V Leiden mutation, 70 percent of those who received treatment had a live birth, but only 44 percent of untreated women had a positive outcome.[51] In another study, researchers were so convinced of the need to treat this disorder that they tested the efficacy of two different doses of heparin instead of evaluating treated versus untreated groups. In their study, women with a history of loss were given either 30 milligrams or 80 milligrams of heparin daily. Live birth rates were 84 percent and 78 percent, respectively.[52]

Factor V Leiden carriers have a higher risk of thromboembolism during pregnancy and throughout their lives.
Left untreated during pregnancy, thrombophilias may pose a threat to the developing baby and the mother. Venous thromboembolism—which occurs when a blood clot formed in a vein travels to other places in the body—occurs eight times as often in pregnant women with inherited thrombophilias as in those without these mutations. One study found that 60 percent of women who develop thromboembolism during pregnancy have one specific mutation: Factor V Leiden.[53]

Outside pregnancy, female Factor V Leiden carriers who take oral contraceptives are at a higher risk for thromboembolism. Researchers disagree about the range of risk; some studies say the risk is ten times that of noncarriers on birth control pills; other studies say the risk could be thirty times greater.[54] Regardless of the exact number, obstetricians will not prescribe the pill to women known to harbor Factor V Leiden. But because testing is so rare, many carriers take oral contraceptives every day, unknowingly putting themselves at greater risk for blood clots.

More than 250,000 cases of venous thromboembolism are diagnosed every year; most cases are older adults, but clots also strike younger people.[55] When clots do develop, 20 to 40 percent of patients carry factor V Leiden; carriers face five- to tenfold greater risk than noncarriers.[56]

Many losses from cervical incompetence could be prevented with better use of cervical measurements and cervical cerclage.

Cervical incompetence—which occurs when the cervix weakens prematurely as pregnancy progresses—is thought responsible for 30 percent of all second-trimester losses.[57] When the weakened cervix can no longer sustain the growing weight of the pregnancy, labor rapidly ensues, resulting in pregnancy loss.

The condition is difficult to diagnose; symptoms resemble other causes of late loss, and there is no reliable diagnostic test. ACOG recommendations tell doctors to wait for a history of *three or more late losses or preterm deliveries* before considering cervical cerclage. The recommendations go on to suggest that (1) women with *two or more* late losses or (2) those with cervical trauma caused by factors such as cone biopsy, a procedure used to treat some cervical cancers, be given serial cervical measurements to monitor for cervical changes during pregnancy.[58]

Doctors use these recommendations differently. Some ignore them, suspecting cervical incompetence after one late loss, refusing to take an unnecessary risk. Others do not take preventive measures until *three late losses—the recommended diagnostic standard*—fating their patients to lose babies that could have been saved.

Many cases of cervical incompetence can be detected before loss by measuring the cervix during pregnancy. A widely accepted study found that at twenty-four weeks gestation, the average cervical length is 35 millimeters. When cervical length is less than 22 millimeters, women face a 20 percent probability of preterm delivery; at less than 15 millimeters, the risk jumps to 33 percent.[59] Another study found that the risk of preterm delivery was 50 percent when the cervix shortened to less than 15 millimeters.[60] Despite these studies and at least ten others that have associated shortened cervical length with increased odds of preterm delivery, many physicians still do not measure cervical length until multiple late losses have occurred. ACOG guidelines acknowledge that cervical ultrasound could help prevent losses after just one late loss; yet when formal treatment recommendations were created, the edict discusses *two or more* late losses before justifying this preventive step.

Once diagnosed, cervical incompetence is treated with bed rest and/or cerclage, stitches placed through the cervix for reinforcement. After cerclage, 80 percent of patients continue the pregnancy to full term.[61] Some physicians combine the two therapies and advise bed rest with a cerclage. In one study of high-risk pregnancies, 44 percent of women who were on bed rest without cerclage delivered preterm, yet none of the women who were given a cerclage and bed rest delivered preterm.[62]

The emergent field of reproductive immunology now offers diagnosis and treatment to women whose losses were previously unexplainable.

Doctors believe that reproductive immunology will bring the most significant advances in preventing pregnancy loss in decades. When women undergo rigorous testing and still get no diagnosis, their losses are said to remain "unexplained." These women should consider further evaluation from a qualified specialist in this emergent field.

Reproductive immunology is the study of how the body's own immune system responds during pregnancy. Our immune system is designed to recognize and attack foreign bodies, battling illness and preserving health. An embryo is technically a foreign object within its mother's body, but instead of attacking, a properly functioning immune system should work to protect the developing embryo. When the natural, protective response does not occur, a patient is said to have an immunological disorder. Many women with unexplained pregnancy loss actually have these treatable conditions, but because the field is so new and limited published research exists, researchers don't know exactly how many. And as is the case with most emerging fields, limited research exists to support some of these therapies.

Dr. Alan E. Beer pioneered the study of reproductive immunology in the 1970s and recently published *Is Your Body Baby-Friendly?*, a book that discusses immune-response problems and the treatments he administered to more than seven thousand couples to overcome these disorders. His average patient was over age thirty-five and had suffered four losses—women to whom mainstream obstetricians offered little hope. With his therapies, many still considered controversial and unproven, more than 85 percent of patients had a live birth.

This field is highly controversial, and patients who seek out these specialists should know that supporting clinical research is still considered limited. Still, any woman who cannot get a diagnosis after loss should know about this developing area of specialization and the encouraging results achieved by most couples.

When bleeding threatens a pregnancy, women should consider bed rest.

The use of bed rest during pregnancy is highly controversial. With the exception of treating cervical incompetence, there is no scientific evidence to support the use of bed rest during pregnancy. However, many high-risk obstetricians still believe that bed rest can help prevent some miscarriages, and they regularly advise at-risk patients to rest.

In his book *Preventing Miscarriage: The Good News*, Dr. Jonathan Scher explains his belief that nature intended women to get more rest during the early stages of pregnancy, hence the fatigue and the frequent nausea. He believes that extra rest can sometimes curb bleeding and prevent miscarriage.

While the value of bed rest to ebb bleeding is considered questionable, from my own experience with bleeding, when I was up more, I bled more. Each woman needs to make this decision for herself, but for me, my body clearly told me that I needed to rest.

Miscarriage can be emotionally devastating.

Women can experience grief, depression, and anxiety after pregnancy loss. Despite their tragic loss, many women do not feel entitled to grieve, especially if the loss was early. Other barriers to grieving are the lack of tangible life or memory, the frequent presence of self-blame, and the inadequacy of support networks.[63] Women generally feel pressure to get "back to normal" before they are ready, often resulting in ongoing psychological distress. Women who do not grieve their loss often suffer longer-lasting psychological, social, and health consequences.[64]

Depression after miscarriage is common. In one study, 35 percent of women reported symptoms of depression soon after miscarriage. Six months after their loss, 26 percent still had symptoms of depression, but only 3 percent had sought psychiatric care.[65] One commonly cited contributor to postloss depression is a lack of emotional support from a spouse or partner.

Anxiety is also a risk. More than twenty studies have linked anxiety and miscarriage, consistently reporting that women who miscarry experience elevated anxiety that usually starts immediately after the loss. The anxiety tends to focus on pregnancy-related issues and generally takes a year to fully subside. Women feel tense, irritable, fatigued, and unable to concentrate or sleep, and report muscle tension.[66]

Couples often believe that the woes of miscarriage will be eased by another pregnancy. For many couples, this is true. But after loss, women battle fear and anxiety during subsequent pregnancies that can make each month tortuous. Three studies have found that pregnant women with a history of loss endure more anxiety during subsequent pregnancies than women without prior miscarriages.[67,68,69]

Pregnancy loss can strain marriages.
Men and women often respond differently to miscarriage. When losses are early, men rarely suffer the anxiety and depression that is so common for their partner. For men, the loss seems less real, and while they care about their spouse's well-being,[70]

many men struggle to be supportive when partners suffer consequences that many husbands just don't understand. This vastly different mark that miscarriage leaves on husbands and wives leads to greater emotional consequences for women, and often harsh consequences for the marriage.

At one year after loss, 32 percent of women report feeling more distant from their husband, and 39 percent say their sexual relationships have suffered.[71] Couples often struggle to close the emotional gap that miscarriage can create when two people experience loss so differently. After loss, couples should consider counseling from a therapist or clergy if the experience strains their relationship.

I also encourage women to seek solace by talking about their loss with supportive friends or family. In our society, miscarriage is still something usually conveyed in whispers, if at all. When women speak to others, they feel less isolated, and quickly discover that their experience is all too common.

The National Institutes of Health does not take the problem of miscarriage seriously, dedicating meager research dollars toward investigating causes of miscarriage.

With nearly a $28 billion budget in 2004, the National Institutes of Health spent just $9.2 million to investigate causes of miscarriage. For a condition that strikes more than two million women every year, miscarriage is among the least funded conditions on a per-capita basis.

Low funding levels are only one indicator that the NIH does not believe miscarriage is a serious disorder that warrants greater focus. The NIH distributes and tracks spending toward 207 health conditions *deemed significant* to public health; *miscarriage is not among the 207 conditions deemed significant enough to track.*

When I contacted the NIH's Office of Research on Women's Health, a division formed in 1990 to "strengthen and enhance research related to diseases, disorders, and conditions that affect women," the office did not know how much money was spent to research causes of miscarriage. A custom report had to be created to answer this question so basic and critical to women's heath.

To further improve obstetric care, more money simply must be directed toward research to prevent miscarriage and preterm birth. Without adequate research dollars, rigorous trials to generate reliable scientific results cannot occur, the pace of care improvements will be impaired, and pregnancies that could have been saved with better care will continue to be lost.

Year	Dollars Spent on Miscarriage Research	Total NIH Research Dollars	Portion of Total NIH Dollars Spent on Miscarriage Research
2000	$5,030,233	$17,820,600,000	0.03 %
2001	$6,753,093	$20,458,100,000	0.03 %
2002	$8,791,374	$23,296,400,000	0.04 %
2003	$9,281,381	$27,066,800,000	0.03 %
2004	$9,168,037	$27,887,500,000	0.03 %

Source: National Institutes of Health, 2005

Twelve states have passed legislation to mandate that insurers cover evaluations after infertility or recurrent pregnancy loss.

Physicians often say that more testing isn't done after pregnancy loss because insurers won't pay for it. In some cases, that is accurate, but this is far from a universal truth. Most insurers follow standard ACOG guidelines, deeming testing "medically unnecessary" until multiple losses have occurred, at which point a limited collection of tests may be covered. But I have seen guidelines from select insurers that do pay for testing before multiple losses, and include some tests not officially recognized by ACOG.

To address the inconsistencies among insurers, the American Society of Reproductive Medicine (ASRM) reports that twelve states have passed legislation that mandates coverage for the diagnosis and treatment of infertility and/or recurrent pregnancy loss. The definitions of infertility and recurrent pregnancy loss vary from state to state, as do the covered treatments. These proactive states are Arkansas, Connecticut, Hawaii, Illinois, Maryland, Massachusetts, Montana, New Jersey, New York, Ohio, Rhode Island, and West Virginia.

Women who live in one of these states can get more detailed information from the ASRM website at http://www.asrm.org/Patients/insur.html or contact their state insurance commissioner's office. I encourage women who live in a state not on this list to contact each of their state representatives and ask how their state is working to secure testing after pregnancy loss.

OBSTETRIC SPECIALTY ORGANIZATIONS THAT OFFER PHYSICIAN REFERRALS

American Society of Reproductive Medicine (ASRM)
ASRM sponsors educational activities for the lay public and continuing medical education for professionals engaged in reproductive medicine. The organization provides information on infertility, menopause, contraception, reproductive surgery, endometriosis, and other reproductive disorders on its website, which allows potential patients to search for a member physician in their city.
http://www.asrm.org

InterNational Council on Infertility Information Dissemination (INCIID)
INCIID, pronounced "inside," has the largest infertility audience worldwide and is a nonprofit dedicated to helping infertile couples find their best family-building options, including treatment

and prevention of pregnancy loss and infertility and guidance for those seeking to adopt. INCIID has developed the first and only IVF scholarship for those with medical and financial need but without insurance to cover the procedure. The organization allows potential patients to search for a member physician in their state. *http://www.inciid.org*

Society for Maternal-Fetal Medicine
The Society for Maternal-Fetal Medicine is the membership organization for obstetricians/gynecologists who have additional formal education and training in maternal-fetal medicine, a specialization involving the diagnosis and treatment of women with complications of pregnancy. The society, which currently has about two thousand active members, allows potential patients to search on its website for a member physician in their state. *http://www.smfm.org*

INFORMATION AND SUPPORT
AFTER PREGNANCY LOSS

March of Dimes

The March of Dimes works to prevent birth defects, premature births, and infant mortality, by funding research, education, and advocacy. Some of the organization's resources are directed toward preventing miscarriage, and their website provides information on causes and prevention of miscarriage and preterm birth, and tests your doctor can complete to screen for preterm labor.

http://www.marchofdimes.com

PreventPregnancyLoss.org

I established this nonprofit organization in 2006 to educate families about preventing pregnancy loss. While several groups exist that are dedicated to fighting infertility and pregnancy loss, I found none whose primary focus was preventing miscarriage, defined as losses before twenty weeks gestation. PreventPregnancyLoss.org

fields outreach efforts to encourage families to consider diagnostic testing after suspicious loss.
http://www.PreventPregnancyLoss.org

RESOLVE: The National Infertility Association
RESOLVE is the oldest and largest consumer nonprofit organization that provides education, advocacy, and support to those struggling with infertility, technically defined as the inability to conceive or carry a pregnancy to term. Most of the organization's resources focus on the inability to conceive, but information is also available about causes of pregnancy loss, treatment options, adoption, and the decision to live child-free, and some of RESOLVE's forty regional offices and local affiliates organize pregnancy loss support groups.
http://www.resolve.org

Share Pregnancy and Infant Loss Support
Share was established to serve those whose lives are touched by the tragedy of pregnancy loss at any gestational age, stillbirth, or the death of a baby in the first few months of life. Share is a national organization with one hundred local chapters where grieving parents can find a supportive, understanding community. The organization also recognizes the difficulty of pregnancy after loss and offers support groups tailored to the needs of these expectant families.
http://www.nationalshareoffice.com

Sidelines National High-Risk Pregnancy Support Network
Sidelines is a nonprofit organization providing international support for women and their families experiencing complicated pregnancies and premature births. The organization offers edu-

cation and a strong support system, matching women with volunteers who have experienced similar problems in past pregnancies. One of the group's specialties is support during bed rest, when women on bed rest are paired with volunteers for e-mail or phone support.
http://www.sidelines.org

Yahoo! Support Groups

As of September 2006, Yahoo! listed 785 support groups under "loss of a child." These groups focus on all ages of loss, including miscarriage and stillbirth.
http://health.dir.groups.yahoo.com/dir/Health___Wellness/Support/ Mourning_and_Loss/Loss_of_Child

Local Hospitals

Check with your local hospital to find a support group for women experiencing complications during pregnancy, or pregnancy loss at any gestational age. Many major medical centers now have a dedicated person whose job consists of organizing and managing support groups. When calling, ask to speak with the person who coordinates support groups.

BOOKS ON EMERGING TREATMENTS TO PREVENT PREGNANCY LOSS

Preventing Miscarriage: The Good News, **by Jonathan Scher, M.D. (2005)**

This is simply the best book on preventing miscarriage that I've ever read. Most of the books on miscarriage fail to go much beyond mainstream care guidelines. Not this one. Dr. Scher provides a broad overview of both established and emerging tests and treatments to prevent pregnancy loss. This book was revised in 2005, but the original version, published in 1990, became my most valued resource when researching causes of my own losses.

Dr. Scher bases his book on published research as well as insights derived from the thousands of patients he has treated at his private Park Avenue practice in New York, where he takes on the most difficult cases and helps most find success. He received national attention in 2004 when he helped a fifty-seven-year-old woman conceive and carry healthy twins to full term.

Is Your Body Baby-Friendly, **by Alan E. Beer, M.D., Julia Kantecki, and Jane Reed (2006)**

Reproductive immunology is a highly specialized and emerging field that offers diagnosis and treatment to couples whose losses remain unexplained, even after a thorough evaluation. Dr. Beer pioneered the study of reproductive immunology, and his book takes a deep dive into the tests and treatments he delivered to more than seven thousand couples. Dr. Beer identified five types of immune system responses that cause reproductive failure, and many infertile couples find that immunotherapy alone can enable them to become parents without IVF. These treatments also help some couples suffering recurrent miscarriage.

Dr. Beer helped thousands of couples, with more than 85 percent of patients delivering healthy babies. His average patient was over age thirty-five, and had endured four prior losses before treatment. While we regrettably lost Dr. Beer in 2006, his important work continues at the Alan E. Beer Center for Reproductive Immunology and Genetics and through the insights shared in his book.

BOOKS ON THE
EMOTIONAL DIFFICULTIES OF
PREGNANCY AFTER LOSS

Pregnancy After a Loss, **by Carol Cirulli Lanham (1999)**
Carol Cirulli Lanham has written a thorough book that helps women prepare, both psychologically and physically, for a new pregnancy after miscarriage, stillbirth, or infant death. The author personally knows the tragedy of pregnancy loss and provides practical considerations for the next pregnancy as well as compassionate understanding of the anxiety inherent in these pregnancies.

Trying Again, **by Ann Douglas and John Sussman, M.D. (2000)**
Ann Douglas and Jon Sussman coauthored this book to lessen the uncertainties about pregnancy and infant loss for parents who have lost a child to miscarriage, stillbirth, or infant loss. They provide facts about pregnancy loss, infant death, and diagnostic testing in an easy-to-read question-and-answer format. The book does a wonderful job of discussing the stress of pregnancy after heartbreaking tragedy.

APPENDIX

More Than 700,000 Women Lose Pregnancies to Treatable Disorders Each Year

Estimated Pregnancies Lost to Treatable Disorders

(Rounded to the nearest thousand)

	Pregnancies and Their Outcomes									
	2000	1999	1998	1997	1996	1995	1994	1993	1992	1991
All Pregnancies	7,875,000	7,714,000	7,676,000	7,606,000	7,646,000	7,649,000	7,817,000	7,986,000	8,129,000	8,172,000
Live Births[1,2]	4,125,000	4,013,000	3,987,000	3,921,000	3,927,000	3,932,000	3,985,000	4,031,000	4,095,000	4,110,000
Induced Abortions[1,2]	1,333,000	1,333,000	1,333,000	1,350,000	1,372,000	1,369,000	1,433,000	1,504,000	1,539,000	1,554,000
Pregnancy Losses[3]	2,417,000	2,368,000	2,356,000	2,335,000	2,347,000	2,348,000	2,399,000	2,451,000	2,495,000	2,508,000
Chromosomally Normal Losses (50% of Pregnancy Losses)										
Normal Losses	1,209,000	1,184,000	1,178,000	1,168,000	1,174,000	1,174,000	1,200,000	1,226,000	1,248,000	1,254,000
Chromosomally Normal Losses with Treatable Disorders (60% of Chromosomally Normal Losses)										
Treatable Losses[4]	725,000	710,000	707,000	701,000	704,000	704,000	720,000	736,000	749,000	752,000

Sources:

1. Ventura, S., Abma, J., Mosher, W., Henshaw, S. *Estimated pregnancy rates for the United States, 1990–2000: an update.* National Vital Statistics Reports, *Vol. 52, no. 23, June 15, 2004.*

2. U.S. Census, 2000.

3. Wilcox, A.J., Weinberg, C.R., O'Connor, J.F., et al. *Incidence of early pregnancy loss.* New England Journal of Medicine. *1988; 319:189–194.*

4. Stephenson, M.D. *Frequency of factors associated with habitual abortion in 197 couples.* Fertility and Sterility. *1996; 66:24–29.*

11. Beer, Alan, M.D. Director and Founder of the Alan E. Beer Center for Reproductive Immunology and Genetics. Interviewed by Darci Klein, May 6, 2005.

12. Owen, J., Yost, N., Berghella, V., et al. Mid-trimester endovaginal sonography in women at high risk for spontaneous preterm birth. *JAMA*. 2001;286: 1340–1348.

13. Harger, J. Cerclage and cervical insufficiency: an evidence-based analysis. *American College of Obstetricians and Gynecologists*. 2002;100:1313–1327.

14. Iams, J., Goldenberg, R., Meis, P., et al. The length of the cervix and the risk of spontaneous premature delivery. *New England Journal of Medicine*. 1996;334: 567–572.

15. Bates, B. Cytogenetic profiles: genetics can triage management of recurrent miscarriage. *OB/GYN News*. July 15, 2004.

16. Theut, S.K., Pedersen, F.A., Zaslow, M.J., Rabinovich, B.A. Pregnancy subsequent to perinatal loss: parental anxiety and depression. *Journal of the American Academy of Child and Adolescent Psychiatry*. 1988;27:289–292.

17. Franche, R.L., Mikail, S.F. The impact of perinatal loss on adjustment to subsequent pregnancy. *Social Science & Medicine*. 1999;48:1613–1623.

18. Cote-Arsenault, D. The influence of perinatal loss on anxiety in multigravidas. *Journal of Obstetric, Gynecologic, and Neonatal Nursing*. 2003;32:623–629.

19. Iams et al. "Length of the cervix."

20. Ibid.

21. Hassan, S., Romero, R., Berry, S. et al. Patients with an ultrasonographic cervical length < or = 15 mm have nearly a 50 percent risk of early spontaneous preterm delivery. *American Journal of Obstetrics and Gynecology*. 2000; 182:1458–1467.

22. O'Brien, J., Hill, A., Barton, J. Funneling to the stitch: an informative ultrasonographic finding after cervical cerclage. *Ultrasound in Obstetrics & Gynecology*. 2002;20:252–255.

23. Vandenbroucke, J., van der Meer, F., Helmerhorst, F., Rosendaal, F. Factor V Leiden: should we screen oral contraceptive users and pregnant women? *BMJ*. 1996;313:1127–1130.

24. Rey, E., Kahn, S., David, M., Shrier, I. Thrombophilic disorders and fetal loss meta-analysis. *Lancet*. 2003;361:901–908.

25. Ginsberg, J., Greer, I., Hirsh, J. Use of antithrombotic agents during pregnancy. *Chest*. 2001;119:122–131.

NOTES

1. NIH research numbers are stated on page 248.
2. American College of Obstetricians and Gynecologists. *Management of Recurrent Early Pregnancy Loss.* Practice Bulletin 24. February 2001.
3. Ibid.
4. Stephenson, M.D. Frequency of factors associated with habitual abortion in 197 couples. *Fertility and Sterility.* 1996; 66:24–29.
5. This estimate is based on 60 percent of chromosomally normal losses with treatable conditions. See the Appendix.
6. National Guideline Clearinghouse. Cervical incompetence. http://www.guidelines.gov; July 1, 2005.
7. Kujovich, J.L. Thrombophilia and pregnancy complications. *American Journal of Obstetrics and Gynecology.* 2004;191:412–424.
8. Ibid.
9. Carp, H., Dolitzky, M., Inbal, A. Thromboprophylaxis improves the live birth rate in women with consecutive recurrent miscarriage and hereditary thrombophilia. *Journal of Thrombosis and Haemostasis.* 2003;1:433–438.
10. Brenner, B., Hoffman, R., Blumenfeld, Z., Weiner, Z., Younis, J. Gestational outcome in thrombophilic women with recurrent pregnancy loss treated by enoxaparin. *Journal of Thrombosis and Haemostasis.* 2000;83:693–697.

26. Grody, W., Griffin, J., Taylor, A., Korf, B., Heit, J. American College of Medical Genetics consensus statement on Factor V Leiden mutation testing. *Genetics in Medicine.* 2001;3:139–148.

27. ACOG. Practice Bulletin 24.

28. Scher, J. *Preventing Miscarriage: The Good News.* New York, NY: HarperCollins; 2005:9.

29. Bates. "Cytogenetic Profiles."

30. Ventura, S., Abma, J., Mosher, W., Henshaw, S. Estimated pregnancy rates for the United States, 1990–2000: an update. *National Vital Statistics Reports,* vol. 52, no. 23. June 15, 2004.

31. ACOG. Practice Bulletin 24.

32. Stephenson, Mary, M.D. Director of the University of Chicago Recurrent Pregnancy Loss Clinic. Interviewed by Darci Klein, August 26, 2005.

33. ACOG. Practice Bulletin 24.

34. Ibid.

35. Stephenson interview, August 26, 2005.

36. Scher. *Preventing Miscarriage.*

37. Bates. "Cytogenetic Profiles."

38. Menasha, J., Levy, B., Hirschhorn, K., Kardon, N. Incidence and spectrum of chromosome abnormalities in spontaneous abortions: new insights from a 12-year study. *Genetics in Medicine.* 2005;7:251–263.

39. Stephenson, M. Management of recurrent early pregnancy loss. *Journal of Reproductive Medicine.* 2006;51:303–310.

40. Bates. "Cytogenetic Profiles."

41. Menasha et al. "Incidence and spectrum of chromosome abnormalities."

42. Stephenson. "Frequency of factors associated with habitual abortion."

43. Scher, Jonathan. Specialist in reproductive immunology in private practice in New York, New York. Interviewed by Darci Klein, September 19, 2006.

44. ACOG. Practice Bulletin 24.

45. Stephenson. "Management of recurrent early pregnancy loss."

46. Kujovich. "Thrombophilia and pregnancy complications."

47. ACOG. Practice Bulletin 24.

48. Kujovich. "Thrombophilia and pregnancy complications."

49. Ibid.

50. Rai, R., Backos, M., Elgaddal, S., Shlebak, A., Regan, L. Factor V Leiden and

recurrent miscarriage—prospective outcome of untreated pregnancies. *Human Reproduction.* 2002;17:442–445.

51. Kujovich. "Thrombophilia and pregnancy complications."

52. Kujovich, J.L. The LIVE-ENOX study: building an enoxaparin bridge over troubled maternal waters. *Journal of Thrombosis and Haemostasis.* 2005;3:779–780.

53. Ginsberg et al. "Use of antithrombotic agents during pregnancy."

54. Spannagl, M., Heinemann, L.A., Schramm, W. Are Factor V Leiden carriers who use oral contraceptives at extreme risk for venous thromboembolism? *European Journal of Contraception and Reproductive Health Care.* 2000;5:105–112.

55. Begelman, S. The Cleveland Clinic. http://www.clevelandclinicmeded.com; March 10, 2006.

56. Kovalevsky, G., Gracia, C., Berlin, J., Sammel, M., Barnhart, K. Evaluation of the association between hereditary thrombophilias and recurrent pregnancy loss. *Archives of Internal Medicine.* 2004;164:558–563.

57. Stray-Pedersen, B., Stray-Pedersen, S. Etiological factors and subsequent reproductive performance in 195 couples with a history of habitual abortion. *American Journal of Obstetrics and Gynecology.* 1984;148:140–146.

58. Harger. "Cerclage and cervical insufficiency."

59. Iams et al. "Length of the cervix."

60. Hassan et al. "Patients with an ultrasonographic cervical length."

61. Scher. *Preventing Miscarriage.*

62. Althuisius, S., Dekker, G., Hummel, P., Bekedam, D., van Geijn, H. Final results of the Cervical Incompetence Prevention Randomized Cerclage Trial (CIPRACT): therapeutic cerclage with bed rest versus bed rest alone. *American Journal of Obstetrics and Gynecology.* 2001;185:1106–1112.

63. Boyce, P.M., Condon, J.T., Ellwood, D.A. Pregnancy loss: a major life event affecting emotional health and well-being. *Medical Journal of Australia.* 2002; 176:250–251.

64. Beutel, M., Deckardt, R., von Rad, M., Weiner, H. Grief and depression after miscarriage: their separation, antecedents, and course. *Psychosomatic Medicine.* 1995;6:517–526.

65. Janssen, HJEM, Cuisinier, M., Hoogduin, KAL, de Graauw, KPHM. Controlled prospective study on the mental health of women following pregnancy loss. *American Journal of Psychiatry.* 1996;153:226–230.

66. Brier, N. Anxiety after miscarriage: a review of the empirical literature and implications for clinical practice. *Birth*. 2004;31:138–142.

67. Theut et al. "Pregnancy subsequent to perinatal loss."

68. Franche and Mikail. "Impact of perinatal loss."

69. Cote-Arsenault. "Influence of perinatal loss on anxiety in multigravidas."

70. Swanson, K.M., Karmali, Z.A., Powell, S.H., Pulvermakher, F. Miscarriage effects on couples' interpersonal and sexual relationships during the first year after loss: women's perceptions. *Psychosomatic Medicine*. 2003;65:902–910.

71. Ibid.